The Forme of Cury, a Roll of Ancient English Cookery, Compiled, About A.D. 1390, by the Master-cooks of King Richard II, and now in the Possession of Gustavus Brander, Esq. A Manuscript of the Editor is Subjoined

# THE FORME OF CURY,

## A ROLL

OF

ANCIENT ENGLISH COOKERY,

Compiled, about A. D. 1390, by the Master-Cooks of King RICHARD II,

Presented afterwards to Queen ELIZABETH, by EDWARD Lord STAFFORD,

And now in the Possession of GUSTAVUS BRANDER, Esq.

Illustrated with NOTES,

And a copious INDEX, or GLOSSARY.

A MANUSCRIPT of the EDITOR, of the same Age and Subject, is subjoined.

BY AN ANTIQUARY.

" ―― ingeniosa gula est." MARTIAL.

LONDON,
PRINTED BY J. NICHOLS.
M DCC LXXX.

T O

GUSTAVUS BRANDER, Efq.
F. R. S. F. S. A. and Cur. Brit. Muf.

SIR,

I RETURN your very curious Roll of Cookery, and I truſt with ſome Intereſt, not full I confeſs nor legal, but the utmoſt which your Debtor, from the ſcantineſs of his ability, can at preſent afford. Indeed, conſidering your reſpectable ſituation in life, and that diffuſive ſphere of knowledge and ſcience in which you are acting, it muſt be exceedingly difficult for any one, how well furniſhed ſoever, completely to anſwer your juſt, or even moſt moderate demands. I intreat the favour of you, however, to accept for once this ſhort payment in lieu of better, or at least as a public testimony of that profound regard wherewith I am,

SIR,

Your affectionate friend,
and most obliged servant,

THE EDITOR.

# PREFACE

TO THE

CURIOUS ANTIQUARIAN READER.

WITHOUT beginning *ab ovo* on a subject so light (a matter of importance, however, to many a modern Catius or Amafinius), by investigating the origin of the Art of Cookery, and the nature of it as practised by the Antediluvians[a]; without dilating on the several particulars concerning it afterwards

[a] If, according to Petavius and Le Clerc, the world was created in autumn, when the fruits of the earth were both plentiful and in the highest perfection, the first man had little occasion for much culinary knowledge roasting or boiling the cruder productions, with modes of preserving those which were better ripened, seem to be all that was necessary for him in the way of *Cury*. And even after he was displaced from Paradise, I conceive, as many others do, he was not permitted the use of animal food [Gen. 1. 29], but that this was indulged to us, by an enlargement of our charter, after the Flood, Gen. ix. 3. But, without wading any further in the argument here, the reader is referred to Gen. ii. 8. feq. iii. 17. feq 23.

amongst the Patriarchs, as found in the Bible [b], I shall turn myself immediately, and without further preamble, to a few cursory observations respecting the Greeks, Romans, Britons, and those other nations, Saxons, Danes, and Normans, with whom the people of this nation are more closely connected.

The Greeks probably derived something of their skill from the East, (from the Lydians principally, whose cooks are much celebrated, [c]) and something from Egypt. A few hints concerning Cookery may be collected from Homer, Aristophanes, Aristotle, &c. but afterwards they possessed many authors on the subject, as may be seen in Athenæus [d]. And as Diætetics were esteemed a branch of the study of medicine, as also they were afterwards [e], so many of those authors were Physicians, and *the Cook* was undoubtedly a character of high reputation at Athens [f].

[b] Genesis xxv. xxvii. Though their best repasts, from the politeness of the times, were called by the simple names of *Bread*, or *a Morsel of bread*, yet they were not unacquainted with modes of dressing meat, boiling, roasting, baking, nor with sauce, or seasoning, as salt and oil, and perhaps some aromatic herbs. Calmet *v. Meats and Eating, and qu. of Honey and cream.* ibid.

[c] Athenæus, lib. xii. cap. 3.

[d] Athenæus, lib. xii. cap. 3. et Casaubon. See also Lister ad Apicium, præf. p. ix. Jungerm. ad Jul. Pollucem, lib. vi. c. 10.

[e] See below. 'Tamen uterque [Torinus et Humelbergius] hæc scripta [i. e. Apicii] ad medicinam vendicarunt.' Lister, præf. p. iv. vii. ix.

[f] Athenæus, p. 519. 660.

As to the Romans; they would of courfe borrow much of their culinary arts from the Greeks, though the Cook with them, we are told, was one of the lowest of their flaves [g]. In the latter times, however, they had many authors on the fubject as well as the Greeks, and the practitioners were men of fome fcience [h], but, unhappily for us, their compofitions are all loft except that which goes under the name of Apicius, concerning which work and its author, the prevailing opinion now feems to be, that it was written about the time of *Heliogabalus* [i], by one *Cælius*, (whether *Aurelianus* is not fo certain) and that *Apicius* is only the title of it [k]. However, the compilation, though not in any great repute, has been feveral times publifhed by learned men.

The Aborigines of Britain, to come nearer home, could have no great expertnefs in Cookery, as they had no oil, and we hear nothing of their butter. They ufed only fheep and oxen, eating neither hares, though fo greatly efteemed at Rome, nor hens, nor geefe, from a notion of fuperftition. Nor did they eat fifh. There was little corn in the interior part of the

[g] Priv. Life of the Romans, p 171. Lifter's Præf. p. iii. but fee Ter An 1 1 Cafaub. ad Jul Capitolin cap 5.

[h] Cafaub ad Capitolin. l c.

[i] Lifter's Præf p ii. vi vii

[k] Fabric Bibl Lat tom. II. p 794. Hence Dr. Bentley ad Hor. ii. ferm. 8. 29. ftiles it *Pfeudapicius*. Vide Lifterum, p iv.

ifland,

island, but they lived on milk and flesh[l]; though it is expresly asserted by Strabo that they had no cheese[m]. The later Britons, however, well knew how to make the best use of the cow, since, as appears from the laws of *Hoel Dda*, A.D. 943, this animal was a creature so essential, so common and useful in Wales, as to be the standard in rating fines, &c.[n].

Hengist, leader of the Saxons, made grand entertainments for king Voitigern[o], but no particulars have come down to us; and certainly little exquisite can be expected from a people then so extremely barbarous as not to be able either to read or write. 'Barbari homines a septentrione, (they are the words 'of Dr. Lister) caseo et ferina subcruda victitantes, 'omnia condimenta adjectiva respuerunt'[p].

Some have fancied, that as the Danes imported the custom of hard and deep drinking, so they likewise introduced the practice of gormandizing, and that this word itself is derived from *Gormund*, the name of that Danish king whom Ælfred the Great per-

---

[l] Cæsar de B. G. v. § 10

[m] Strabo, lib iv p 200. Pegge's Essay on Coins of Cunob, p 95.

[n] Archæologia, iv p 61 Godwin, de Præsul p 596 seq.

[o] Mat. 5 p 9 Gaufr Mon. vi. 12.

[p] Lister ad Apic. p xi where see more to the same purpose

suaded

[ v ]

suaded to be christened, and called Æthelstane [q]. Now 'tis certain that Hardicnut stands on record as an egregious glutton [r], but he is not particularly famous for being a *curious Viander*; 'tis true again, that the Danes in general indulged excessively in feasts and entertainments [s], but we have no reason to imagine any elegance of Cookery to have flourished amongst them. And though Guthrum, the Danish prince, is in some authors named *Gormundus* [t]; yet this is not the right etymology of our English word *Gormandize*, since it is rather the French *Gourmand*, or the British *Gormod* [u]. So that we have little to say as to the Danes.

I shall take the later English and the Normans together, on account of the intermixture of the two nations after the Conquest, since, as lord Lyttelton observes, the English accommodated themselves to the Norman manners, except in point of temperance in eating and drinking, and communicated to them their own habits of drunkenness and immoderate feasting [x]. Erasmus also remarks, that the English in his time

---

[q] Spelm. Life of Ælfred, p 66, Drake, Eboracum. Append. p civ

[r] Speed's History.

[s] Monf. Mallet, cap. 12.

[t] Wilkins, Concil I. p. 204 Drake, Ebor. p 316. Append. p civ cv.

[u] Menage, Orig. v. Gourmand.

[x] Lord Lyttelton, Hist. of H. II. vol. iii. p. 49.

were

[ vi ]

were attached to *plentiful and splendid tables*, and the same is observed by Harrison [y]. As to the Normans, both William I. and Rufus made grand entertainments [z]; the former was remarkable for an immense paunch, and withal was so exact, so nice and curious in his repasts [a], that when his prime favourite William Fitz-Osberne, who as steward of the household had the charge of the Cury, served him with the flesh of a crane scarcely half-roasted, he was so highly exasperated, that he lifted up his fist, and would have strucken him, had not Eudo, appointed *Dapifer* immediately after, warded off the blow [b].

*Dapifer*, by which is usually understood *steward of the king's household* [c], was a high officer amongst the Normans, and *Larderarius* was another, clergymen

---

[y] Harrison, Descript. of Britain, p. 165, 166.

[z] Sor, p. 102. 128.

[a] Lord Lyttelton observes, that the Normans were delicate in their food, but without excess. Life of Hen. II. vol III. p. 47.

[b] Dugd. Bar. I. p. 109. Henry II. served to his son. Lord Lyttelton, IV. p. 298.

[c] Godwin de Præsul. p. 695, renders *Carver* by *Dapifer*, but this I cannot approve. See Thoroton p. 23. 28. Dugd. Bar. I. p. 441. 620. 109. Lib. Nig. p. 342. Kennet Par. Ant. p. 119. And, to name no more, Spelm. in voce. The *Carver* was an officer inferior to the *Dapifer*, or *Sewara*, and even under his control. Vide Leic. Collect. VI. p. 2. And yet I find Sir Walter Manny when young was carver to Philippa queen of king Edward III. Barnes Hist. of E. III. p. 171. The *Steward* had the name of *Dapifer*, I apprehend, from serving up the first dish. V. supra

then

[ vii ]

then often occupying this post, and sometimes made bishops from it [d]. He was under the *Dapifer*, as was likewise the *Cocus Dominicæ Coquinæ*, concerning whom, his assistants and allowances, the *Liber Niger* may be consulted [e]. It appears further from *Fleta*, that the chief cooks were often providers, as well as dressers, of victuals [f]. But *Magister Coquinæ*, who was an esquire by office, seems to have had the care of pourveyance, A. D. 1340 [g], and to have nearly corresponded with our *clerk of the kitchen*, having authority over the cooks [h]. However, the *Magnus Coquus, Coquorum Præpositus, Coquus Regius*, and *Grans Queux*, were officers of considerable dignity in the palaces of princes; and the officers under them, according to Du Fresne, were in the French court A. D. 1385, much about the time that our Roll was made, ' Queus, Aideurs, Asteurs, Paiges, Souffleurs, ' Enfans, Sauffiers de Commun, Sauffiers devers le ' Roy, Sommiers, Poulliers, Huiffiers' [i].

In regard to religious houses, the Cooks of the greater foundations were officers of consequence,

[d] Sim Dunelm col 227 Hoveden, p. 469 Malmf de Pont. p 286.

[e] Lib. Nig Scaccarii, p. 347.

[f] Fleta, II cap. 75

[g] Du Fresne, v. Magister.

[h] Du Fresne, ibid.

[i] Du Fresne, v. Coquus. The curious may compare this List with Lib. Nig. p 347.

though

though under the Cellarer [k], and if he were not a monk, he nevertheless was to enjoy the portion of a monk [l]. But it appears from Somner, that at Christ Church, Canterbury, the *Lardyrer* was the first or chief cook [m], and this officer, as we have seen, was often an ecclesiastic. However, the great Houses had Cooks of different ranks [n], and manors and churches [o] were often given *ad cibum* and *ad victum monachorum* [p]. A fishing at Lambeth was allotted to that purpose [q]. But whether the Cooks were Monks or not, the *Magistri Coquinæ*, Kitcheners, of the monasteries, we may depend upon it, were always monks, and I think they were mostly ecclesiastics elsewhere: thus when Cardinal Otto, the Pope's legate, was at Oxford, A. 1238, and that memorable fray happened between his retinue and the students, the *Magister Coquorum* was the Legate's brother, and was there

[k] In Somner, Ant. Cant Append p 36 they are under the *Mafr Coquinæ*, whose office it was to purvey, and there again the chief cooks are proveditors, different usages might prevail at different times and places But what is remarkable, the *Coquinariu*, or Kitcherer, which seems to answer to *Magifri Coquinæ*, is placed before the Cellarer in Tanner's Notitia, p. xxx. but this may be accidental

[l] Du Fresne, v. Coquus.
[m] Somner, Append p. 36
[n] Somner, Ant Cant. Append. p. 36.
[o] Somner, p 41.
[p] Somner, p. 36, 37. 39, sæpius.
[q] Somner l. c.

killed.

killed [r]. The reason given in the author, why a person so nearly allied to the Great Man was assigned to the office, is this, 'Ne procuraretur aliquid vene-'norum, quod nimis [i. e. valde] timebat legatus,' and it is certain that poisoning was but too much in vogue in these times, both amongst the Italians and the good people of this island [s], so that this was a post of signal trust and confidence. And indeed afterwards, a person was employed to *taste*, or *take the assaie*, as it was called [t], both of the messes and the water in the ewer [u], at great tables, but it may be doubted whether a particular person was appointed to this service, or it was a branch of the *Sewer's* and cup-bearer's duty, for I observe, the *Sewer* is sometimes called *Prægustator* [x], and the cup-bearer tastes the water elsewhere [y]. The religious houses, and their presidents, the abbots and priors, had their days of *Gala*, as likewise their halls for strangers, whom, when persons of rank, they often entertained with splendour and magnificence. And as for the secular clergy, archbishops and bishops, their feasts,

[r] M Paris, p4. 69

[s] Dugd Bar. I p 45. Stow, p. 184 M. Paris, p. 377. 517. M Westm p 364

[t] Lel. Collectan. VI. p. 7. seq.

[u] Ibid p 9 13

[x] Compare Leland, p 3 with Godwin de Præsul. p 695. and so Junius in Etymol. v. Sewer.

[y] Leland, p 8, 9. There are now *two yeomen of the mouth* in the king's houschold.

[ x ]

of which we have some upon record [z], were so superb, that they might vie either with the regal entertainments, or the pontifical suppers of ancient Rome (which became even proverbial [a]), and certainly could not be dressed and set out without a large number of Cooks [b]. In short, the satirists of the times before, and about the time of, the Reformation, are continually inveighing against the high-living of the bishops and clergy, indeed luxury was then carried to such an extravagant pitch amongst them, that archbishop Cranmer, A. 1541, found it necessary to bring the secular clergy under some reasonable regulation in regard to the furnishing of their tables, not excepting even his own [c].

After this historical deduction of the *Ars coquinaria,* which I have endeavoured to make as short as possible, it is time to say something of the Roll which

---

[z] That of George Neville, archbishop of York, 6 Edw. IV. and that of William Warham, archbishop of Canterbury, A D. 1504. These were both of them inthronization feasts. Leland, Collectan. V 7 p. 2 and 6 of Appendix. They were wont *munere sanguinem* after these superb entertainments, p. 32.

[a] Hor. l. I. Od xiv 28. where see Monsf Dacier.

[b] Sixty-two were employed by archbishop Neville And the hire of cooks at archbishop Warham's feast came to 23 l. 6 s. 8 d

[c] Strype, Life of Cranmer, p. 451. or Lel Coll ut supra, p. 38. Sumptuary laws in regard to eating were not unknown in ancient Rome Erasm Colloq p 81 ed Schrev. nor here formerly, see Len. Col VI. p 36. for 5 Ed. II.

[ xi ]

is here given to the public, and the methods which the Editor has purfued in bringing it to light.

This vellum Roll contains 196 *formulæ*, or recipes, and belonged once to the earl of Oxford [d]. The late James Weſt eſquire bought it at the Earl's ſale, when a part of his MSS were diſpoſed of, and on the death of the gentleman laſt mentioned it came into the hands of my highly-eſteemed friend, the preſent liberal and moſt communicative poſſeſſor. It is preſumed to be one of the moſt ancient remains of the kind now in being, riſing as high as the reign of king Richard II. [e]. However, it is far the largeſt and moſt copious collection of any we have; I ſpeak as to thoſe times. To eſtabliſh its authenticity, and even to ſtamp an additional value upon it, it is the identical Roll which was preſented to queen Elizabeth, in the 28th year of her reign, by lord Stafford's heir, as appears from the following addreſs, or inſcription, at the end of it, in his own hand-writing. ' Antiquum hoc monumentum oblatum et miſ-
' ſum eſt majeſtati veſtræ viceſimo ſeptimo die menſis
' Julij, anno regni veſtri fæliciſſimi viceſimo viij ab

---

[d] I preſume it may be the ſame Roll which Mr Hearne mentions in his Lib. Nig. Scaccarii, I. p 346. See alſo three different letters of his to the earl of Oxford, in the Brit. Muſ. in the ſecond of which he ſtiles the Roll *a piece of antiquity, and a very great rarity indeed.* Harl. MSS. N° 7523.

[e] See the Proem.

' humi-

'humilimo vestro subdito, vestræq majestati fidelissimo
'E. Stafford,
'Hæres domus subversæ Buckinghamiens.' [f]

The general observations I have to make upon it are these: many articles, it seems, were in vogue in the fourteenth century, which are now in a manner obsolete, as cranes, curlews, herons, seals [g], porpoises, &c. and, on the contrary, we feed on sundry fowls which are not named either in the Roll, or the Editor's MS. [h] as quails, rails, teal, woodcocks, snipes, &c. which can scarcely be numbered among the *small birds* mentioned 19. 62. 154.[i]. So as to fish, many species appear at our tables which are not found in the Roll, trouts, flounders, herrings, &c.[k]. It were easy and obvious to dilate here on the variations of taste at different periods of time, and the reader would probably not dislike it; but so many other particulars demand our attention, that I shall content myself with observing in general, that where-

[f] This lord was grandson of Edward duke of Buck., beheaded A. 1521, whose son Henry was restored in blood, and this Edward, the grandson, born about 1571, might be 14 or 15 years old when he presented the Roll to the Queen.

[g] Mr Topham's MS. has *seas* among the fish, and see archbishop Nevil's Feast, 6 E IV. to be mentioned below.

[h] Of which see an account below.

[i] See Northumb. Book, p. 107, and Notes.

[k] As to carps, they were unknown in England t. R. II. Fuller, Worth. in Suffolk. p. 58. 113. Stow, Hist. 1058.

as a very able *Italian* critic, *Latinus Latinius*, passed a sinister and unfavourable censure on certain seemingly strange medlies, disgusting and preposterous messes, which we meet with in *Apicius*; Dr. *Lister* very sensibly replies to his strictures on that head, ' That these messes are not immediately to be rejected,
' because they may be displeasing to some. *Plutarch*
' testifies, that the ancients disliked *pepper* and the
' sour juice of lemons, insomuch that for a long time
' they only used these in their wardrobes for the sake
' of their agreeable scent, and yet they are the most
' wholesome of all fruits. The natives of the *West*
' *Indies* were no less averse to *salt*, and who would
' believe that *hops* should ever have a place in our
' common beverage[1], and that we should ever think
' of qualifying the sweetness of malt, through good
' housewifry, by mixing with it a substance so egre-
' giously bitter? Most of the *American* fruits are ex-
' ceedingly odoriferous, and therefore are very dif-
' gusting at first to us *Europeans* on the contrary, our
' fruits appear insipid to them, for want of odour.
' There are a thousand instances of things, would
' we recollect them all, which though disagreeable to
' taste are commonly assumed into our viands, indeed,
' *custom* alone reconciles and adopts sauces which are
' even nauseous to the palate *Latinus Latinius* there-

[1] The Italians still call the hop *ertiwa uba* There was a petition against them t. H VI Fuller, Worth. p 317, &c Evelyn, Sylva, p. 201. 469. ed. Hunter.

' fore

'fore very rashly and absurdly blames *Apicius*, on
'account of certain preparations which to him, for-
'sooth, were disrelishing [m]. In short it is a known
maxim, that *de gustibus non est disputandum*,

And so Horace to the same purpose:

'Tres mihi convivæ prope dissentire videntur,
'Poscentes vario multum diversa palato.
'Quid dem? quid non dem? renuis tu quod jubet
  'alter.
'Quod petis, id sane est invisum acidumque
  'duobus.

Hor. II. Epist. ii.

And our Roll sufficiently verifies the old observation
of Martial — *ingeniosa gula est*.

Our Cooks again had great regard to the eye, as
well as the taste, in their compositions; *flourishing*
and *strewing* are not only common, but even leaves of
trees gilded, or silvered, are used for ornamenting
messes, see N° 175 [n]. As to colours, which perhaps
would chiefly take place in suttleties, blood boiled
and fried (which seems to be something singular)
was used for dying black, 13. 141. saffron for yel-

---

[m] Lister Præf. ad Apicium, p. xi.

[n] So we have *leaves of gold* Lel. Collect IV p. 227. and a
wild boar's head *gilt*. p. 294. A peacock with *gilt reb*. VI. p. 6.
*Leb. Lambart gilt*, ibid.

low, and fanders for red°. Alkenet is alfo ufed for colouring P, and mulberries q, amydon makes white, 68, and turnefole ʳ *pownas* there, but what this colour is the Editor profeffes not to know, unlefs it be intended for another kind of yellow, and we fhould read *jownas*, for *jaulnas*, orange-tawney. It was for the purpofe of gratifying the fight that *fotiltees* were introduced at the more folemn feafts. Rabelais has comfits of an hundred colours.

Cury, as was remarked above, was ever reckoned a branch of the Art Medical; and here I add, that the verb *curare* fignifies equally to drefs victuals ˢ, as to cure a diftemper, that every body has heard of *Doctor Diet, kitchen phyfick*, &c. while a numerous band of medical authors have written *de cibis et alimentis*, and have always claffed diet among the *non-naturals*; fo they call them, but with what propriety they beft know. Hence Junius ' Δίαιτα Græcis eft ' victus, ac fpeciatim certa victûs ratio, qualis a *Medicis* ad tuendam valetudinem præfcribitur ᵗ.' Our

---

° N° 68. 20. 58 See my friend Dr Percy on the Northumberland-Book, p. 415 and MS Ed. 34.

ᴾ N° 47. 51 84.

q N° 93. 132. MS Ed 37.

ʳ Perhaps Turmerick See ad loc.

ˢ Ter Andr I 1. where Donatus and Mad Dacier explain it of Cooking. Mr Hearne, in defcribing our Roll, fee above, p xi, by an unaccountable miftake, read *Fay* inftead of *Cury*, the plain reading of the MS

ᵗ Junii Etym. v. Diet.

Cooks

[ xvi ]

Cooks exprefsly tell us, in their proem, that their work was compiled 'by affent and avyfement of 'maifters of phifik and of philofophie that dwellid 'in his [the King's] court' where *phyfik* is ufed in the fenfe of medecine, *phyficus* being applied to perfons profeffing the Art of Healing long before the 14th century [u], as implying *fuch* knowledge and fkill in all kinds of natural fubftances, conftituting the *materia medica*, as was neceffary for them in practice. At the end of the Editor's MS is written this rhyme,

Explicit coquina que eft optima medicina [x].

There is much relative to eatables in the *Schola Salernitana*; and we find it ordered, that a phyfician fhould over-fee the young prince's wet-nurfe at every meal, to infpect her meat and drink [y].

But after all the avyfement of phyficians and philofophers, our proceffes do not appear by any means to be well calculated for the benefit of recipients, but rather inimical to them. Many of them are fo highly feafoned, are fuch ftrange and heterogeneous

[u] Reginaldus Phificus. M Paris, p. 410. 412. 573 764 Et in Vit. p 94. 103 Chaucer's Medc's is a doctor of phifick, p. 4. V. Junii Etym. voce Phyfician For later times, v J Roftus, p 93.

[x] That of Donatus is more modeft 'Culina medicinæ famulatrix 'eft'

[y] Lel Collect IV p 183 'Diod. Siculus refert primos Ægypti Reges victum quotidianum omnino fumpfiffe ex medicorum præfcripto.' Lifter au Apic. p ix.

compositions, meer olios and gallimawfreys, that they seem removed as far as possible from the intention of contributing to health, indeed the messes are so redundant and complex, that in regard to herbs, in N° 6, no less than ten are used, where we should now be content with two or three and so the sallad, N° 76, consists of no less than 14 ingredients. The physicians appear only to have taken care that nothing directly noxious was suffered to enter the forms. However, in the Editor's MS. N° 11, there is a prescription for making a *colys*, I presume a *cullis*, or invigorating broth, for which see Dodsley's Old Plays, vol. II. 124. vol. V. 148. vol. VI. 355. and the several plays mentioned in a note to the first mentioned passage in the Edit. 1780 [z].

I observe further, in regard to this point, that the quantities of things are seldom specified [a], but are too much left to the taste and judgement of the cook, who, if he should happen to be rash and inconsiderate, or of a bad and undistinguishing taste, was capable of doing much harm to the guests, to invalids especially.

Though the cooks at Rome, as has been already noted, were amongst the lowest slaves, yet it was not so more anciently; Sarah and Rebecca cook, and so

---

[z] See also Lylie's Euphues, p 282. Cavendish, Life of Wolsey, p. 151, where we have *callis*, malè; Cole's and Lyttleton's Dict. and Junii Etymolog. v Collice

[a] See however, N° 191, and Editor's MS II. 7.

do Patroclus and Automedon in the ninth Iliad. It were to be wished indeed, that the Reader could be made acquainted with the names of our *master-cooks*, but it is not in the power of the Editor to gratify him in that, this, however, he may be assured of, that as the Art was of consequence in the reign of Richard, a prince renowned and celebrated in the Roll [b], for the splendor and elegance of his table, they must have been persons of no inconsiderable rank: the king's first and second cooks are now esquires by their office, and there is all the reason in the world to believe they were of equal dignity heretofore [c]. To say a word of king *Richard* he is said in the proeme to have been ' acōnted the best and ryalleft vyānd [cu-' riofo in eating] of all efté kynges.' This, however, must rest upon the testimony of our cooks, since it does not appear otherwise by the suffrage of history, that he was particularly remarkable for his niceness and delicacy in eating, like Heliogabalus, whose favourite dishes are said to have been the tongues of peacocks and nightingales, and the brains of parrots and pheasants [d], or like Sept. Geta, who, according to Jul. Capitolinus [e], was so curious, so whimsical, as to order the dishes at his dinners to consist of things which all began with the same letters. Sardanapalus

[b] Vide the proeme.

[c] See above.

[d] Univ. Hist. XV p 352 ' Æsopus pater linguas avium huma-
' na vocales lingua cænavit, filius margaritas.' Lifter ad Apicium,
p vii.

[e] Jul. Capitolinus, c. 5.

again,

[ xix ]

again, as we have it in Athenæus[f], gave a *præmium* to any one that invented and served him with some novel cate, and Sergius Orata built a house at the entrance of the Lucrine lake, purposely for the pleasure and convenience of eating the oysters perfectly fresh. Richard II is certainly not represented in story as resembling any such epicures, or capriccioso's, as these[g]. It may, however, be fairly presumed, that good living was not wanting among the luxuries of that effeminate and dissipated reign.

My next observation is, that the messes both in the Roll and the Editor's MS, are chiefly soups, potages, ragouts, hashes, and the like hotche-potches, entire joints of meat being never *served*, and animals, whether fish or fowl, seldom brought to table whole, but hacked and hewed, and cut in pieces or gobbets[h], the mortar also was in great request, some messes being actually denominated from it, as *mortrews*, or *mortercl)s*, as in the Editor's MS. Now in this state of things, the general mode of eating must either have been with the spoon or the fingers; and this perhaps may have been the reason that spoons be-

[f] Athenæus, lib xii c. 7 Something of the same kind is related of Heliogabalus, Lister Præf ad Apic. p vii.

[g] To omit the paps of a pregnant sow, Hor I. Ep xv 40. where see Monf Dacier, Dr Lister relates, that the tongue of carps were accounted by the ancient Roman palate men most delicious meat Worth. in Sussex. See other instances of extravagant Roman luxury in Lister's Præf to Apicius, p. vii

[h] See, however, N° 33, 34, 35. 146.

d 2 came

came an usual present from gossips to their god-children at christenings[i]; and that the bason and ewer, for washing before and after dinner, was introduced, whence the *ewarer* was a great officer[k], and the *ewery* is retained at Court to this day[l], we meet with *damasse water* after dinner[m], I presume, perfumed, and the words *ewer*, &c. plainly come from the Saxon *eƿe*, or French *eau*, *water*.

Thus, to return, in that little anecdote relative to the Conqueror and William Fitz-Osbern, mentioned above, not the crane, but *the flesh of the crane* is said to have been under-roasted. Table, or case knives, would be of little use at this time[n], and the art of carving is perfectly useless, as to be almost unknown. In about a century afterwards, however, as appears from archbishop Nevile's entertainment, many articles were served whole, and lord Wylloughby was the carver[o]. So that carving began now to be prac-

---

[i] The king, in Shakespeare, Hen VIII act v. sc 2 and 3, calls the gifts of the sponsors, *spoons*. These were usually gilt, and, the figures of the apostles being in general carved on them, were called *apostle spoons*. See Mr. Steevens's note in Ed. 1778, vol VII p 312 and Gent Mag 1768 p 426.

[k] Lel Collect IV p. 328. VI. p 2.

[l] See Dr Percy's curious notes on the Northumb. Book, p. 417.

[m] Ibid. VI p 5. 18.

[n] They were not very common at table among the Greeks Casaub. ad Athenæum, col 278 but see Lel Coll VI p 7

[o] Leland, Collectan. VI p. 2 Archbishop Warham also had his carver, ibid p. 18. See also, IV. p. 236. 240. He was a great officer. Nor Lumb. Book, p. 443.

tised,

[ xxi ]

tifed, and the proper terms devifed. Wynken de Worde printed a *Book of Kervinge*, A. 1508, wherein the faid terms are regiftered ᵖ. ' The ufe of *forks* ' at table, fays Dr. Percy, did not prevail in Eng- ' land till the reign of James I. as we learn from a ' remarkable paffage in *Coryat* ᵠ', the paffage is indeed curious, but too long to be here tranfcribed, where brevity is fo much in view; wherefore I fhall only add, that forks are not now ufed in fome parts of Spain ʳ. But then it may be faid, what becomes of the old Englifh hofpitality in this cafe, the *roaft-beef of Old England*, fo much talked of? I anfwer, thefe bulky and magnificent difhes muft have been the product of later reigns, perhaps of queen Elizabeth's time, fince it is plain that in the days of Rich. II. our anceftors lived much after the French fafhion. As to hofpitality, the houfeholds of our Nobles were immenfe, officers, retainers, and fervants, being entertained almoft without number; but then, as appears from the Northumberland Book, and afterwards from the houfehold eftablifhment of the prince of Wales, A. 1610, the individuals, or at leaft fmall parties, had their *quantum*, or ordinary, ferved out, where any good œconomy was kept, apart to themfelves ˢ. Again, we find in our Roll, that great quan-

---

ᵖ Ames, Typ Ant. p. 90. The terms may alfo be feen in Rand, Holme III. p 78.

ᵠ Dr Percy, l c.

ʳ Thickneffe, Travels, p. 260.

ˢ Dr. Birch, Life of Henry prince of Wales, p. 457, feq.

tives of the respective viands of the hashes, were often made at once, as N° 17, *Take hernes or conynges.* 24, *Take haris.* 29, *Take pygges.* And 31, *Take gees*, &c. So that hospitality and plentiful house-keeping could just as well be maintained this way, as by the other of cumbrous unwieldy messes, as much as a man could carry.

As the messes and sauces are so complex, and the ingredients consequently so various, it seems necessary that a word should be spoken concerning the principal of them, and such as are more frequently employed, before we pass to our method of proceeding in the publication.

Butter is little used. 'Tis first mentioned N° 81, and occurs but rarely after[t]; 'tis found but once in the Editor's MS, where it is written *boter*. The usual substitutes for it are oil-olive and lard, the latter is frequently called *grece*, or *grece*, or *whitegrece*, as N° 18. 193. *Capons in Greace* occur in Birch's Life of Henry prince of Wales, p 459, 460. and see Lye in Jun Etym. v. *Greasie*. Bishop Patrick has a remarkable passage concerning this article: 'Though we read of cheese in *Homer*, *Euripides*, '*Theocritus*, and others, yet they never mention '*butter* nor hath Aristotle a word of it, though he 'hath sundry observations about cheese for butter

[t] N° 91, 92 160.

[ xxiii ]

'was not a thing then known among the *Greeks*;
'though we see by this and many other places, it was
'an ancient food among the eastern people [u].' The
Greeks, I presume, used oil instead of it, and butter
in some places of scripture is thought to mean only
cream [x].

Cheese. See the last article, and what is said of
the old Britons above; as likewise our Glossary.

Ale is applied, N° 113, et alibi, and often in the Editor's MS. as 6, 7, &c. It is used instead of wine, N° 22,
and sometimes along with bread in the Editor's MS. [y]
Indeed it is a current opinion that brewing with hops
was not introduced here till the reign of king
Henry VIII. [z] *Bere*, however, is mentioned A.
1504 [a].

Wine is common, both red, and white, N° 21. 53.
37. This article they partly had of their own growth [b],
and partly by importation from France [c] and Greece [d].

[u] Bishop Patrick on Genesis xviii 8
[x] Calmet, v Butter So Judges iv 19. compared with v 25.
[y] II N° 13, 14, 15
[z] Stow, Hist p. 1038
[a] Lel Coll VI p 30 and see Dr. Percy on Northumb. Book, p 414.
[b] Archæologia, I. p. 319 III p 53.
[c] Barrington's Observ. on Statutes, p 209 252. Edit 3d Archæolog I p. 330 Fitz-Stephen, p 33 Lel. Coll. VI. p. 14. Northumb. Book, p. 6 and notes.
[d] N° 20, 64. 99.

They

They had alfo Rhenifh [e], and probably feveral other forts. The *vynegreke* is among the fweet wines in a MS of Mr. Aftle.

Rice. As this grain was but little, if at all, cultivated in England, it muft have been brought from abroad. Whole or ground-rice enters into a large number of our compofitions, and *refmolle*, N° 96, is a direct preparation of it.

Alkenet. *Anchufa* is not only ufed for colouring, but alfo fried and yfondred, 62. yfondyt, 162. i. e. diffolved, or ground. 'Tis thought to be a fpecies of the *buglos*.

Saffron. Saffrum, Brit. whence it appears, that this name ran through moft languages. Mr. Weever informs us, that this excellent drug was brought hither in the time of Edward III.[f] and it may be true; but ftill no fuch quantity could be produced here in the next reign as to fupply that very large confumption which we fee made of it in our Roll, where it occurs not only as an ingredient in the proceffes, but alfo is ufed for colouring, for flourifhing or garnifhing. It makes a yellow, N° 68, and was imported from Egypt, or Cilicia, or other parts of the Levant, where the Turks call it Safran, from the Arabic Zapheran,

[e] N° 99.
[f] Fun. Mon. p 624.

whence the English, Italians, French, and Germans, have apparently borrowed their respective names of it. The Romans were well acquainted with the drug, but did not use it much in the kitchen [g]. Pere Calmet says, the Hebrews were acquainted with anise, ginger, saffron, but no other spices [h].

**Pynes.** There is some difficulty in enucleating the meaning of this word, though it occurs so often. It is joined with dates, N° 20. 52. with honey clarified, 63. with powder-fort, saffron, and salt, 161. with ground dates, raisins, good powder, and salt, 186. and lastly they are fried, 38. Now the dish here is *morree*, which in the Editor's MS. 37, is made of mulberries (and no doubt has its name from them), and yet there are no mulberries in our dish, but pynes, and therefore I suspect, that mulberries and pynes are the same, and indeed this fruit has some resemblance to a pyne-cone. I conceive *pynnonade*, the dish, N° 51, to be so named from the pynes therein employed; and quære whether *pyner* mentioned along with powder-fort, saffron, and salt, N° 155, as above in N° 161, should not be read *pynes*. But, after all, we have cones brought hither from Italy full of nuts, or kernels, which upon roasting come out of their *capsulæ*, and are much eaten by the common people, and these perhaps may be the thing intended.

[g] Dr Lister, Præf. ad Apicium, p. xii.
[h] Calmet. Dict. v. Eating.

Honey was the great and univerſal ſweetner in remote antiquity, and particularly in this iſland, where it was the chief conſtituent of *mead* and *metheglin*. It is ſaid, that at this day in *Paleſtine* they uſe honey in the greateſt part of their ragouts[i]. Our cooks had a method of clarifying it, N° 18. 41. which was done by putting it in a pot with whites of eggs and water, beating them well together, then ſetting it over the fire, and boiling it; and when it was ready to boil over to take it and cool it, N° 59. This I preſume is called *clere honey*, N° 151. And, when honey was ſo much in uſe, it appears from Barnes that *refining* it was a trade of itſelf[k].

Sugar, or Sugur[l], was now beginning here to take place of honey, however, they are uſed together, N° 57. Sugar came from the Indies, by way of Damaſcus and Aleppo, to Venice, Genoa, and Piſa, and from theſe laſt places to us[m]. It is here not only frequently uſed, but was of various ſorts, as *cypre*, N° 41. 99. 120. named probably from the iſle of Cyprus, whence it might either come directly to us, or where it had received ſome improvement by way of refining. There is mention of *blanch powder or*

---

[i] Calmet Dict. v Meats.
[k] Barnes, Hiſt. of E III. p 111.
[l] N° 70. Edi or' MS 17. a ibi.
[m] Moll, Geogr. II. p 130. Harris, Coll of Voyages, I. p. 874. Ed. Campbell.

*white*

[ xxvii ]

*white sugar*, 132. They, however, were not the same, for see N° 193. Sugar was clarified sometimes with wine [n].

Spices. *Species*. They are mentioned in general N° 133, and *whole spices*, 167, 168. but they are more commonly specified, and are indeed greatly used, though being imported from abroad, and from so far as Italy or the Levant (and even there must be dear), some may wonder at this but it should be considered, that our Roll was chiefly compiled for the use of noble and princely tables, and the same may be said of the Editor's MS. The spices came from the same part of the world, and by the same route, as sugar did. The *spicery* was an ancient department at court, and had its proper officers.

As to the particular sorts, these are,

Cinamon. *Canell* 14. 191. *Canel*, Editor's MS. 10. *Kanell*, ibid. 32. is the Italian *Canella*. See Chaucer. We have the flour or powder, N° 20. 62. See Wiclif. It is not once mentioned in Apicius.

Macys, 14. 121. Editor's MS. 10. *Maces*, 134. Editor's MS. 27. They are used whole, N° 158. and are always expressed plurally, though we now use the singular, *mace*. See Junii Etym.

[n] N° 20. 148.

Clove.

[ xxviii ]

Cloves. N° 20. Dishes are flourished with them, 22. 158. Editor's MS. 10. 27. where we have *clowys gylofres*, as in our Roll, N° 194. *Powdour gylofre* occurs 65. 191. Chaucer has *clowe* in the singular, and see him v. Clove-gelofer.

Galyngal, 30. and elsewhere. Galangal, the long rooted cyperus[o], is a warm cardiac and cephalic. It is used in powder, 30. 47. and was the chief ingredient in *galentine*, which, I think, took its name from it.

Pepper. It appears from Pliny that this pungent, warm seasoning, so much in esteem at Rome[p], came from the East Indies[q], and, as we may suppose, by way of Alexandria. We obtained it no doubt, in the 14th century, from the same quarter, though not exactly by the same route, but by Venice or Genoa. It is used both whole, N° 35, and in powder, N° 83. And long-pepper occurs, if we read the place rightly, in N° 191.

Ginger, gyngyn. 64. 136. alibi. Powder is used, 17. 20. alibi. and Rabelais IV. c. 59. the white

---

[o] Glossary to Chaucer. See the Northumb. Book, p 415 and 19. also Quincy's Dispens and Brookes's Nat. Hist. of Vegetables.

[p] Lister, Præf ad Apicium, p xii.

[q] Plinius, Nat. Hist. XII. cap 7.

powder,

powder, 131. and it is the name of a mess, 139. quære whether *gyngyn* is not misread for *gyngyr*, for see Junii Etym. The Romans had their ginger from Troglodytica [r].

Cubebs, 64. 121. are a warm spicy grain from the east.

Grains of Paradice, or *de parys*, 137.[s] are the greater cardamoms.

Noix muscadez, 191. nutmegs.

The caraway is once mentioned, N° 53. and was an exotic from *Caria*, whence, according to Mr. Lye, it took its name: 'sunt semina, inquit, *carri* vel *carret*, 'sic dicti a Caria, ubi copiosissimè nascitur [t].'

Powder-douce, which occurs so often, has been thought by some, who have just peeped into our Roll, to be the same as sugar, and only a different name for it; but they are plainly mistaken, as is evident from 47. 51. 164. 165. where they are mentioned together as different things. In short, I take powder-douce to be either powder of galyngal, for see Editor's MS II. 20. 24, or a compound made of sundry

[r] Bochart. III. col 332
[s] See our Gloss, voce Greynes.
[t] Lye, in Junii Etymolog.

aromatic

[ xxx ]

aromatic spices ground or beaten small, and kept always ready at hand in some proper receptacle. It is otherwise termed *good powders*, 83. 130. and in Editor's MS 17. 37. 38 [u]. or *powder* simply, N° 169, 170. *White powder-douce* occurs N 51, which seems to be the same as blanch-powder, 132. 193. called *blaynshe powder*, and bought ready prepared, in Northumb. Book, p. 19. It is sometimes used with powder-fort, 38. 156. for which see the next and last article.

Powder fort, 10. 11. seems to be a mixture likewise of the warmer spices, pepper, ginger, &c. pulverized: hence we have *powder-fort of gynger, other of carel*, 14. It is called *strong powder*, 22. and perhaps may sometimes be intended by *good powders*. If you will suppose it to be kept ready prepared by the vender, it may be the *powder marchant*, 113. 118 found joined in two places with powder-douce. This Speght says is what gingerbread is made of, but Skinner disapproves this explanation, yet, says Mr. Urry, gives none of his own.

After thus travelling through the most material and most used ingredients, the *spykenard ae spayn* occurring only once, I shall beg leave to offer a few words on the nature, and in favour of the present publication, and the method employed in the prosecution of it.

[u] B. see the next article.

The

## ffor to make chalkmenny

Take þe chese and of flessh of capons· or of henny & hakke smal and grynde hem smalle in a morter w{i}t{h} mylke of almands w{i}t{h} þe broth of freyssh beef· or freyssh flessh· & put the flessh i{n} þ{e} mylke o{n} i{n} broth and set he{m} to þe fyre· & take hem w{i}t{h} flo{ur} of ryse· or saffron· or anyson· as chargeant as þ{e} blan{c} desire· & w{i}t{h} zolks of ayren and safron for to make h{i}t zelow· and when it is dressit in dyssh{es} blank desir{e} styk aboue clow{es} so gilofre· & strawe poudre of sugur gale aboue· and ser it forth·

[ xxxi ]

The common language of the *formulæ*, though old and obsolete, as naturally may be expected from the age of the MS, has no other difficulty in it but what may easily be overcome by a small degree of practice and application[x]. however, for the further illustration of this matter, and the satisfaction of the curious, a *fac simile* of one of the recipes is represented in the annexed plate. If here and there a hard and uncouth term or expression may occur, so as to stop or embarrass the less expert, pains have been taken to explain them, either in the annotations under the text, or in the Index and Glossary, for we have given it both titles, as intending it should answer the purpose of both[y]. Now in forming this alphabet, as it would have been an endless thing to have recourse to all our glossaries, now so numerous, we have confined ourselves, except perhaps in some few instances, in which the authorities are always mentioned, to certain contemporary writers, such as the Editor's MS, of which we shall speak more particularly hereafter, Chaucer, and Wiclif; with whom we have associated Junius' Etymologicon Anglicanum.

[x] Doing, hewing, hacking, grynding, kerving, &c. are easily understood.

[y] By combining the Index and Glossary together, we have had an opportunity of elucidating some terms more at large than could conveniently be done in the notes. We have also cast the Index to the Roll, and that to the Editor's MS, into one alphabet, distinguishing, however, the latter from the former.

[ xxxii ]

As the abbreviations of the Roll are here retained, in order to eſtabliſh and confirm the age of it, it has been thought proper to adopt the types which our printer had projected for Domeſday-Book, with which we find that our characters very nearly coincide.

The names of the diſhes and ſauces have occaſioned the greateſt perplexity. Theſe are not only many in number, but are often ſo horrid and barbarous, to our ears at leaſt, as to be inveloped in ſeveral inſtances in almoſt impenetrable obſcurity. Biſhop Godwin complains of this ſo long ago as 1616[z]. The *Contents* prefixed will exhibit at once a moſt formidable liſt of theſe hideous names and titles, ſo that there is no need to report them here. A few of theſe terms the Editor humbly hopes he has happily enucleated, but ſtill, notwithſtanding all his labour and pains, the argument is in itſelf ſo abſtruſe at this diſtance of time, the helps ſo few, and his abilities in this line of knowledge and ſcience ſo ſlender and confined, that he fears he has left the far greater part of the taſk for the more ſagacious reader to ſupply: indeed, he has not the leaſt doubt, but other gentlemen of curioſity in ſuch matters (and this publication is intended for them alone) will be ſo happy as to clear up ſeveral difficulties, which appear now to him inſuperable. It muſt be confeſſed again, that

---

[z] Godwin de Præſul. p. 684.

[ xxxiii ]

the Editor may probably have often failed in those very points, which he fancies and flatters himself to have elucidated, but this he is willing to leave to the candour of the public.

Now in regard to the helps I mentioned; there is not much to be learnt from the Great Inthronization-feast of archbishop Robert Winchelsea, A. 1295, even if it were his; but I rather think it belongs to archbishop William Warham, A. 1504[a]. Some use, however, has been made of it.

Ralph Bourne was installed abbot of St. Augustine's, near Canterbury, A 1309, and William Thorne has inserted a list of provisions bought for the feast, with their prices, in his Chronicle[b].

The Great Feast at the Inthronization of George Nevile archbishop of York, 6 Edward IV. is printed by Mr. Hearne[c], and has been of good service.

[a] In Dr. Drake's edition of archbishop Parker, p lxiii it is given to archbishop Winchelsea but see Mr. Battely's Append. to Cantuaria Sacra, p 27. or the Archæologia, I p 350 and Leland's Collectanea, VI p. 30. where it is again printed, and more at large, and ascribed to Warham

[b] Thorne, Chron inter X Script. Col. 2010 or Lel. Collect. VI p 34 Ed 1770

[c] Leland, Collect. VI p 2 See also Randle Holme, III p 77 Bishop Godwin de Præsul p 695 Ed Richardson, where there are some considerable variations in the messes or services, and he and the Roll in Leland will correct one another.

f          Elizabeth,

[ xxxiv ]

Elizabeth, queen of king Henry VII was crowned A. 1487, and the messes at the dinner, in two courses, are registered in the late edition of Leland's Collectanea, A. 1770 [d], and we have profited thereby.

The Lenten Inthronization-feast of archbishop William Warham, A. 1504 [e], given us at large by Mr. Hearne [f], has been also consulted.

There is a large catalogue of viands in Rabelais, lib. iv. cap. 59. 60. And the English translation of Mr. Ozell affording little information, I had recourse to the French original, but not to much more advantage.

There is also a Royal Feast at the wedding of the earl of Devonshire, in the Harleian Misc. N° 279, and it has not been neglected.

Randle Holme, in his multifarious *Academy of Armory*, has an alphabet of terms and dishes [g]; but though I have pressed him into the service, he has not contributed much as to the more difficult points.

The Antiquarian Repertory, vol. II. p. 211, exhibits an entertainment of the mayor of Rochester, A. 1460; but there is little to be learned from thence. The present work was printed before N° 31 of the Antiquarian Repertory, wherein some ancient recipes in Cookery are published, came to the Editor's hand.

[d] Vol IV p. 226.
[e] See first paragraph before
[f] Leland's Collect VI. p. 16.
[g] Holme, Acad. of Armory, III. p. 81.

I must

I muſt not omit my acknowledgments to my learned friend the preſent dean of Carliſle, to whom I ſtand indebted for his uſeful notes on the Northumberland-Houſehold Book, as alſo for the book itſelf.

Our chief aſſiſtance, however, has been drawn from a MS belonging to the Editor, denoted, when cited, by the ſignature *MS Ed.* It is a vellum miſcellany in ſmall quarto, and the part reſpecting this ſubject conſiſts of ninety-one Engliſh recipes (or *nyms*) in cookery. Theſe are diſpoſed into two parts, and are intituled, ' Hic incipiunt univerſa ſervicia tam de ' carnibus quam de piſſibus.'[h] The ſecond part, relates to the dreſſing of fiſh, and other lenten fare, though forms are alſo there intermixed which properly belong to fleſh-days. This leads me to obſerve, that both here, and in the Roll, meſſes are ſometimes accommodated, by making the neceſſary alterations, both to fleſh and fiſh-days.[i] Now, though the ſubjects of the MS are various, yet the hand writing is uniform, and at the end of one of the tracts is added, ' Explicit maſſa Compoti, Anno Dñi M<sup>lo</sup> CCC<sup>mo</sup> ' octogeſimo primo ipſo die Felicis et Audacti.'[k] i.e. 30 Aug. 1381, in the reign of Rich. II. The language and orthography accord perfectly well with this date, and the collection is conſequently contemporary with our Roll, and was made chiefly, though

---

[h] It is *piſſbus* again in the title to the Second Part.

[i] N° 7. 84. here N° 17 55 97.

[k] In the common calendars of our miſſals and breviaries, the latter ſaint is called *Adavctus*, but in the Kalend. Roman of Joh. Fronto, Paris 1652, p 126, he is written *Audaſtus*, as here; and ſee Martyrolog Bedæ, p 414.

[ xxxvi ]

not altogether, for the use of great tables, as appears from the *surgeon*, and the great quantity of venison therein prescribed for.

As this MS is so often referred to in the annotations, glossary, and even in this preface, and is a compilation of the same date, on the same subject, and in the same language, it has been thought adviseable to print it, and subjoin it to the Roll, and the rather, because it really furnishes a considerable enlargement on the subject, and exhibits many forms unnoticed in the Roll.

To conclude this tedious preliminary detail, though unquestionably a most necessary part of his duty, the Editor can scarcely forbear laughing at himself, when he reflects on his past labours, and recollects those lines of the poet Martial;

Turpe est difficiles habere nugas,

Et stultus labor est ineptiarum. II. 86.

and that possibly mesdames *Cutte* and *Raffald*, with twenty others, might have far better acquitted themselves in the administration of this province, than he has done. He has this comfort and satisfaction, however, that he has done his best, and that some considerable names amongst the learned, Humelbergius, Torinus, Bethius, our countryman Dr Lister, Almeloveen, and others, have bestowed no less pains in illustrating an author on the same subject, and scarcely of more importance, the *Pseudo-Apicius*.

# THE

# FORME OF CURY.

---

... fome ᵃ of cury ᵇ was compiled of the chef Maiſt Coḳ of kyng Richard the Secunde kyng of . nglond ᶜ aftır the Conqueſt. the which was acoñted þ̇ ᵈ beſt and ryalleſt vyand ᵉ of alle cſtē . yng̊ ᶠ and it was cōpiled by aſſent and

---

ᵃ This is a kind of Preamble to the Roll. A ſpace is left for the initial word, intended to be afterwards written in red ink, and preſumed to be Đis. Fome, the lineola over it being either caſually omitted, or ſince obliterated, means form, written Fóme below, and in Nº 195.

ᵇ Cury. Cookery. We have adopted it in the Title. V. Preface.

ᶜ ynglond. E was intended to be prefixed in red ink. Vide Note ᵃ and ᶠ.

ᵈ þ. This Saxon letter with the power of *th*, is uſed almoſt perpetually in our Roll and the Editor's Mſ. Every one may not have adverted to it, but this character is the ground of our preſent abbreviations y̓ the, y̓ that, ẙ this, &c. the y in theſe caſes being evidently only an altered and more modern way of writing þ.

ᵉ vyānd. This word is to be underſtood in the concrete, *quaſi* vyander, a curious epicure, an *Apicius*. V Preface

ᶠ cſtē ynges. Chriſtian kings. *K* being to be inſerted afterwards (v. note ᵃ and ᶜ) in red ink. Chaucer, v. chriſten.

A  avyſe-

[ 2 ]

avɣſement of Maiſters and ᵍ phiſik ʰ and of philoſophie þat dwellid in his court. Firſt it techiþ a man for to make cōmune potages and cōmune meetis for howſhold as þeɣ ſhold be made craftly and holſomly. Aftirward it techiþ for to make curious potages ⁊ meet and ſotiltees ⁱ for alle manē of States bothe hye and lowe. And the techyng of the fōme of making of potages ⁊ of meet bothe of fleſsh and of fifsh. buth ᵏ y ſette here by noumbre and by ordre. ſſo þis little table here ſewyng ˡ wole teche a man with oute taryyng꞉ to fynde what meete þ̄ hym luſt for to have.

or ᵐ to make gronden benes. . . . . . . . . I.
F or to make drawen benes. . . . . . . . . II.
f or to make grewel forced. . . . . . . . . III.
C aboches in potage. . . . . . . . . . . . IIII.
r apes in potage. . . . . . . . . . . . . . V.
E owt of Fleſsh . . . . . . . . . . . . . . VI.

ᵍ and Read *of*
ʰ Phiſik V. Preface
ⁱ Soſtlees Devices in paſte, wax, and confectionary ware; reviving now, in ſome meaſure, in our grander deſerts. V. Index.
ᵏ buth *Be*, or *are*. V Index
ˡ ſewing. Following, from the French Hence our *enſue* written formerly *enſu* Skelton, p 144, and *enſiew*, Ames Typ. Ant p, 9.
ᵐ F is omitted for the reaſon given in note ᵃ.

hebolas.

[ 3 ]

hebolas . . . . . . . . . . . . . . . . . . . . VII.
Gowid in potage. . . . . . . . . . . . . . . VIII.
ryſe of Fleſsh. . . . . . . . . . . . . . . . . IX.
Funges. . . . . . . . . . . . . . . . . . . . . . X.
burſen. . . . . . . . . . . . . . . . . . . . . . XI.
Corat. . . . . . . . . . . . . . . . . . . . . . XII.
noumbles. . . . . . . . . . . . . . . . . . . XIII.
Roobroth. . . . . . . . . . . . . . . . . . . . XIIII.
tredure. . . . . . . . . . . . . . . . . . . . . XV.
Monchelet. . . . . . . . . . . . . . . . . . . XVI.
bukkenade. . . . . . . . . . . . . . . . . . . XVII.
Connat . . . . . . . . . . . . . . . . . . . . . XVIII.
drepee. . . . . . . . . . . . . . . . . . . . . XIX.
Mawmenee. . . . . . . . . . . . . . . . . . XX.
egurdouce. . . . . . . . . . . . . . . . . . . XXI.
Capons in Concy. . . . . . . . . . . . . . . XXII.
haares in talbotes. . . . . . . . . . . . . . XXIII.
Haares in papdele. . . . . . . . . . . . . . XXIIII.
connyng in Cynee. . . . . . . . . . . . . . XXV.
Connyng in gravey. . . . . . . . . . . . . . XXVI.
*Chykens in gravey. . . . . . . . . . . . . . XXVII.
filet in galyntyne. . . . . . . . . . . . . . . XXVIII.
Pigges in ſawſe ſawge. . . . . . . . . . . XXIX.
ſawſe madame. . . . . . . . . . . . . . . . XXX.
Gees i hoggepot. . . . . . . . . . . . . . . XXXI.
carnel of pork . . . . . . . . . . . . . . . . XXXII.

A 2 Chikens

[ 4 ]

C hikens in Caudell. . . . . . . . . . . . xxxiii.

c hikens in hocchee. . . . . . . . . . xxxiiii.

F or to boyle Fesānt, Partyches } . . . xxx.v.
    Capons and Curlewes. . . }

b lank manng. . . . . . . . . . . . . . . . xxxvi.

B lank Defforre. . . . . . . . . . . . . xxxvii.

m orree . . . . . . . . . . . . . . . . . . xxxviii.

C harlet. . . . . . . . . . . . . . . . . xxxix.

c harlet y forced . . . . . . . . . . . xx. ii.

C awdel ferry. . . . . . . . . . . . . . . . xx. ii. i.

i ufshell. . . . . . . . . . . . . . . . . . xx. ii iii.[n]

I ufshell enforced. . . . . . . . . . . xx. ii. iiii.

m ortrews. . . . . . . . . . . . . . . . xx. ii. v.

B lank mortrews. . . . . . . . . . . . . xx. ii. vi.

b rewet of almony. . . . . . . . . . . xx. ii. vii.

P eions y ftewed. . . . . . . . . . . xx. ii. viii.

I ofeyns. . . . . . . . . . . . . . . . xx. ii. ix.

T artlet. . . . . . . . . . . . . . . . . xx. ii. x.

p ynnonade. . . . . . . . . . . . . . . . xx. ii xi.

R ofee. . . . . . . . . . . . . . . . . . xx ii xii.

c ormarye. . . . . . . . . . . . . . . . xx. ii. xiii.

N ew noumbl of Deer. . . . . . . . . xx. ii xiiii.

n ota. . . . . . . . . . . . . . . . . . xx ii. xv.

N ota. . . . . . . . . . . . . . . . . . xx. ii xvi.

i pynee. . . . . . . . . . . . . . . . . xx. ii. xvii.

[a] N° xx. ii. ii. is omitted.

Chyryfe.

[ 5 ]

Chyryſe . . . . . . . . . . . . . . . . . xx. II. XVIII.
payn Fōndewe . . . . . . . . . . . . xx. II XIX.
Crotoñ . . . . . . . . . . . . . . . . . . xx. III.
vyne grace . . . . . . . . . . . . . . . xx. III. I.
Fonnell . . . . . . . . . . . . . . . . . xx. III. II.
douce ame . . . . . . . . . . . . . . . xx. III. III.
Connyng in Cirypp . . . . . . . . xx. III. IIII.
leche lumbard . . . . . . . . . . . . xx. III. V.
Connyng in clere broth . . . . . . xx. III. VI.
payn Ragoñ . . . . . . . . . . . . . . xx. III. VII.
Lete lard . . . . . . . . . . . . . . . . xx. III. VIII.
furmente with porpeys . . . . . . xx. III. IX.
Perrey of Pesōn . . . . . . . . . . . xx. III. X.
pesōn of Almayn . . . . . . . . . . xx. III. XI.
Chiches . . . . . . . . . . . . . . . . . xx. III. XII.
frenche owt . . . . . . . . . . . . . . xx. III. XIII.
Makke . . . . . . . . . . . . . . . . . . xx. III. XIIII.
a quapat . . . . . . . . . . . . . . . . xx. III. XV.
Salat . . . . . . . . . . . . . . . . . . . xx. III. XVI.
fenkel in ſopp . . . . . . . . . . . . xx. III. XVII.
Clat . . . . . . . . . . . . . . . . . . . . xx. III. XVIII.
appulmoy . . . . . . . . . . . . . . . xx. III. XIX.
Slete ſopp . . . . . . . . . . . . . . . xx. IIII.
letelorye . . . . . . . . . . . . . . . . xx. IIII. I.
Sowp Dorry . . . . . . . . . . . . . xx. IIII. II.
rapey . . . . . . . . . . . . . . . . . . xx. IIII. III.

Sauſe

[ 6 ]

| | xx | |
|---|---|---|
| S aufe Sarzyne............ | IIII. | IIII. |
| c̛ reme of almãnd.......... | xx IIII. | V. |
| G rewel of almãnd......... | xx IIII. | VI. |
| c̛ awdel of almand mylk...... | xx IIII. | VII. |
| I ow̛t of almãnd mylk....... | xx IIII. | VIII. |
| f ygey............... | xx IIII. | IX. |
| P ochee.............. | xv IIII. | X. |
| b rewet of ayren.......... | xx IIII. | XI. |
| M acrows............. | xx IIII. | XII. |
| t oftee.............. | xx IIII. | XIII. |
| G yndawdry............ | xx IIII. | XIIII. |
| e rbowle............. | xx IIII. | XV. |
| R efmolle............. | xx IIII. | XVI. |
| v yannde Cipre.......... | xx IIII. | XVII. |
| V yande Cipre of Samon..... | xx IIII. | XVIII. |
| v yande Ryal........... | xx IIII. | IX. |
| C ompoft............. | | c. |
| g elee of Fyfsh.......... | | c I. |
| G elee of flefsh.......... | | c. II. |
| C hyfanne............ | | c. III. |
| c. ongur in fawce........ | | c. IIII. |
| R ygh in fawce.......... | | c. V. |
| m akerel in fawce......... | | c. VI. |
| P ykes in brafey......... | | c VII. |
| p orpeys in broth......... | | c. VIII. |
| B allck broth........... | | c. IX. |

eles

e les in brewet. . . . . . . . . . . . . . c. x.
C awdel of Samōn. . . . . . . . . . c. xi.
p lays in Cynee. . . . . . . . . . . . . c. xii.
F or to make Flaumpeyns. . . . . . c. xiii.
f or to make noumbl⁹ in lent. . . . . . c. xiiii.
F or to make Chawdōn for lent. . . . . c. xv.
f urmente with porpays. . . . . . . . c. xvi.
F ylett⁹ in galyntyne. . . . . . . . . . . c. xvii.
v eel in buknade. . . . . . . . . . . . . c. xviii.
S ool⁹ in Cyney. . . . . . . . . . . . . . c. ix.
t ench⁹ in Cyney. . . . . . . . . . . . . xx vi.
O yſters in gravey. . . . . . . . . . . xx vi. i.
m uſkels in brewet. . . . . . . . . . . xx vi. ii.
O yſters in Cyney. . . . . . . . . . . . xx vi. iii.
c awdel of muſkels. . . . . . . . . . . . xx vi. iiii.
M ortrews of Fyſh. . . . . . . . . . . xx vi. v.
l aumpreys in galyntyne. . . . . . . xx vi. vi
L aumproñs in galyntyne. . . . . . . xx vi. vii.
l oſyns in Fyſhe day. . . . . . . . xx vi. viii.
S owp⁹ in galyntyne. . . . . . . . . xx vi. ix.
f obre ſawſe. . . . . . . . . . . . . xx vi. x.
C olde Brewet. . . . . . . . . . . . . xx vi. xi.
p eer⁹ in confyt. . . . . . . . . . . xx vi. xii.
E gur douce of Fyſh. . . . . . . . xx vi. xiii.
C old Brewet. . . . . . . . . . . . xx vi. xiiii.
P evorat for Veel and Venyſoñ . . . vi. xv.

ſawce

[ 8 ]

ſawce blanche for Capons y ſode. . . . VI. XVI.
Sawce Noyre for Capons y roſted. . . . VI. XVII.
galentyne. . . . . . . . . . . . . . . VI. XVIII.
Gyngen. . . . . . . . . . . . . . . VI. XIX.
verde ſawſe. . . . . . . . . . . . . VII.
Sawce Noyre for malard. . . . . . VII. I.
cawdel for Gees. . . . . . . . . . VII. II.
Chawdon for Swann. . . . . . . . VII. III.
ſawce Camelyne. . . . . . . . . . VII. IIII.
Lumbard Muſtard. . . . . . . . . VII. V.
nota. . . . . . . . . . . . . . . . VII. VI.
Nota. . . . . . . . . . . . . . . . VII. VII.
fryto blanched. . . . . . . . . . VII. VIII.
Fryto of paſtnak. . . . . . . . . VII. IX.
fryto of mylke. . . . . . . . . . VII. X.
fryto of Erbes. . . . . . . . . . VII. XI.
raiſiowls. . . . . . . . . . . . . VII. XII.
Whyte milat. . . . . . . . . . . VII. XIII.
cruſtard of fleſsh. . . . . . . . . VII. XIIII.
Mylat of Pork. . . . . . . . . . VII. XV.
cruſtard of Fyſsh. . . . . . . . . VII. XVI.
Cruſtard of erbis on fyſsh day. . . VII. XVII.
leſsh fryed in lenton. . . . . . . VII. XVIII.
Waſtels y farced. . . . . . . . . VII. XIX.
ſawge y farced. . . . . . . . . . VIII.
Sawgeat . . . . . . . . . . . . VIII. I.

cryſpes.

[ 9 ]

| | |
|---|---|
| c ryſpes. | XX VIII. II. |
| C ryſpels. | XX VIII. III. |
| t artee. | VIII. IIII. |
| T art in Ymbre day. | XX VIII. V. |
| t art de Bry. | XX VIII VI. |
| T art de Brymlent. | XX VIII. VII. |
| t art of Fleſh | XX VIII. VIII. |
| T artlet. | XX VIII. IX. |
| t art of Fyſh. | XX VIII. X. |
| S ambocade. | XX VIII. XI. |
| e ibolat. | VIII. XII. |
| N yſebek. | XX VIII. XIII. |
| f or to make Pō Dorı yes. & oþe þyng. | XX VIII. XIIII. |
| C otagr. | XX VIII. XV. |
| h art rows. | XX VIII. XVI. |
| P otews. | XX VIII. XVII. |
| f achus. | VIII. XVIII. |
| B urſews. | XX VIII XIX. |
| f pynoch y fryed. | XX IX. |
| B enes y fryed. | XX IX. I. |
| r uſhews of Fruyt. | XX IX. II. |
| D aryols. | IX. III. |
| f laumpens. | XX IX IIII. |
| C hewet on fleſh day. | XX V. |
| c hewet on fyſh day. | XX IX VI. |
| H aſtelet. | XI. VII. |

B          comadoȓ

c omadoȓ. . . . . . . . . . . . . . . . xx. IX. VIII.
C haſtletꝯ. . . . . . . . . . . . . . . . xx IX. IX.
f or to make twey pecys of Fleſshe } . . xx IX. X.
    to faſten to gydre. . . . .
p ur fait y pocras. . . . . . . . . . . . xx. IX. XI.
F or to make blank manḡ. . . . . . . xx IX. XII.
f or to make Blank Deſue. . . . . . xx IX. XIII.
F or to make mawmoune. . . . . . . xx IX XIIII.
t he pety puānt. . . . . . . . . . . . xx IX. XV.
A nd the pete puant. . . . . . . . . xx IX. XVI.

## 𝔛plicit tabula.

For to make gronden Benes [a].        I.

TAKE benes and dry hē ī a noſt [b] or in an Ovene and hulle hē wele and wyndewe [c] out þ hulk and wayſhe hē clene ā do hē to ſeeþ in gode broth [d] ā ete hē w' Bacon.

For to make drawen Benes.        II.

Take benes and ſeeþ hē and grynde hem ī a morť [e] and drawe hem up [f] w' gode broth ā do Oynons in the broth grete mynced [g] ā do þ to and colo it with Safron and ſerve it forth.

---

[a] Gronden Benes. Beans ground (y grōnd, as N° 27 53. 105.) ſtript of their hulls. This was a diſh of the poorer houſeholder, as alſo is 4 and 5, and ſome others.

[b] a noſt. An oſt, or kiln. Vide Gloſſ. *voce* Oſt.

[c] wyndewe. Winnow.

[d] gode broth  Prepared beforehand.

[e] mort'  Mortar

[f] drawen hem up.  Mix them.

[g] grete mynced.  Groſsly, not too ſmall.

[ 12 ]

#### For to make grewel forced ʰ. III.

Take grewel and do to the fyre with gode flefsh and feeþ it wel take the lire ⁱ of Pork and grynd it fmal ᵏ and drawe the grewel thurgh a Stynoʳ ˡ and coloʳ it wiþ Safron and ſue ᵐ forth.

#### Caboches ⁿ in Potage. IIII.

Take Cabochʳ and quart hē and feeth hem in gode broth with Oynons ȝ mynced and the whyte of Lekes y flyt and corue fmale ᵒ and do þ to fafron ā falt and force it w powdō douce ᵖ.

#### Rapes ᵠ in Potage. V.

Take rapus and make hē clene and waifsh hē clene. quare hem ʳ. pboile hē. take hem up. caft hem in a gode broth and feeþ hē. mynce Oynons and caft þ to

---

ʰ forced, farced, enriched with flefh. Vide Glofſ.
ⁱ lre Flefh
ᵏ grynd it fmal Bruife or beat in a mortar.
ˡ ſty o' Strainer
ᵐ ſue. Serve Vide Glofſ
ⁿ Cabocher. Probably caborges.
ᵒ corue ſmale Cut fmall V. corue in Glofſ
ᵖ po co douce. Sweet aromatic powder V Pref.
ᵠ Rapes, or rapus Turnips.
ʳ Quarlon Cut them in ſquares, or fmal pieces. V. Glofſ

Safron

[ 13 ]

Safroñ and Salt and meſſe it forth with powdo� douce.
In the wiſe ˢ make of Paſturnak̃ ᵗ and skyrwat ᵘ.

### Eowt ˣ of Flesh. VI.

Take Borage. cool ʸ. langdebef ᶻ. pſel ᵃ. bet. orage ᵇ. auance ᶜ. violet ᵈ. ſaẃay ᵉ. and fenkel ᶠ. and whane þey buth ſode: preſſe hem wel ſmale. caſt hem in gode broth ā ſeeþ hē. and ſūe hem forth.

### Hebolace ᵍ. VII.

Take Oynoñs and erbes and hewe hem ſmall and do þ̃ to gode broth. and aray ʰ it as þ̃ dideſt caboch̃.

---

ˢ in the wiſe, *i. e* in the ſame manner. *Self* or *ſame*, ſeems to be caſually omitted. Vide Nº 11 and 122.

ᵗ Paſturnakes, for parſnips or carrots. V. Gloſſ.

ᵘ ſkyrwates, for ſkirrits or ſkirwicks.

ˣ Eowtes Lowtes, Nº 88, where, in the proceſs, it is *Rowtes*. Quære the meaning, as Roots does not apply to the matter of the Recipe. In Nº 73 it is written *owtes*    ʸ Cole, or colewort.

ᶻ Langdebef. Bugloſs, bugloſſum ſylveſtre Theſe names all ariſe from a ſimilitude to an ox's tongue. V Mſ Ed. Nº 43.

ᵃ Peiſel. Parſley

ᵇ orage Orach, *Atriplex*. Miller, Gard. Dict.

ᶜ auance. Fortè Avens. V Avens, in Gloſſ

ᵈ The leaves probably, and not the flower.

ᵉ Savory.   ᶠ Fenkel. Fennil.

ᵍ Hebolace Contents, Hebolas, for *Herbolas*, from the herbs uſed, or, if the firſt letter be omitted (ſee the Contents), *Chebolas*, from the Chibols employed.

ʰ aray. Dreſs, ſet it out.

If

If þey be in fyſsh day. make [i] on the ſame manē [k] wiþ waī and oyle. and if it be not in Lent alye [l] it with zolkes of Eyren [m]. and dreſſe it forth and caſt þꝫ to powdoꝛ douce.

### Gourdes in Potage. VIII.

Take young Gowrdꝫ pare hem and kerue [n] hem on pecys. caſt hem in gode broth. and do þꝫ to a gode ptye [o] of Oynōs mynced. take Pork ſoden grynd it and alye it þ w and wiþ zolkes of ayreīn. do þꝫ to ſafron and ſalt. and meſſe it forth with powdoꝛ douce.

### Ryſe [p] of Fleſh. IX.

Take Ryſe and waiſhe hem clene. and do hē in erthen pot with gode broth and lat hem ſeeþ wel. afterward take Almand mylke [q] and do þꝫ to. and coloꝛ it wiþ ſafron ā ſalt. ā meſſe forth.

### Funges [r]. X.

Take Funges and pare hem clene and dyce hem [s]. take leke and ſhred hym ſmall and do hȳ to ſeeþ

---

[i] make. Dreſs. Vide Gloſſ.  [k] manē. manner.
[l] alye. Mix. V. Gloſſ.  [m] Eyren. Eggs. V Gloſſ.
[n] kerve. Cut  [o] ptye. Party, i. e. quantity.
[p] Ryſe. Rice. V Gloſſ.  [q] Almand mylke. V. Gloſſ.
[r] Funges. Muſhrooms
[s] dyce hem. Cut them in ſquares  Vide quare in Gloſſ.

in gode broth. colo͝ur it with fafron and do p̄ inne powdo͝ur fort ᵗ.

### Burfen ᵘ. XI.

Take the whyte of Lek̄. flype hem and fhrede hem fmall. take Noumbl͝es ˣ of fwyne and p̄boyle hem in broth and wyne. take hym up and dreffe hȳ and do the Leke in the broth. feeþ and do the Noumbl͝es p̄ to make a Lyo͝ur ʸ of brode blode and vynegre and do p̄ to Powdo͝ur fort feeþ Oyno͞ns mynce hem and do p̄ to. the felf wife make of Pigg͝es.

### Corat ᶻ. XII.

Take the Noumbl͝es of Calf. Swyne. or of Shepe. p̄boile hem and fkerne hem to dyce ᵃ. caft hem in gode broth and do p̄ to erbes. grynde chyball ᵇ. fmale y hewe. feeþ it tendre and lye it with zolkes of eyren͞. do p̄ to v'ious ᶜ fafron powdo͝ur douce and falt. and fue it forth.

---

ᵗ Powdo͝ur fort. Vide Preface
ᵘ Burfen. Qu. the etymon.
ˣ Noumbles. Entrails. V. Gloff.
ʸ Lyo', Lyour. A mixture. Vide *alye* in Gloff.
ᶻ Corat Qu.
ᵃ kerve hem to dyce. V. *quare* in Gloff.
ᵇ Chyballes Chibols, young onions. V. Gloff.
ᶜ v'ious. Verjuice.

Noumbles.

## Noumbles. XIII.

Take noumblˀ of Deer oþ ᵈ of oþ beeſt pboile hem kerf hem to dyce. take the ſelf broth or better. take brede and grynde with the broth. and temp it ᵉ up with a gode qntite of vyneḡ and wyne. take the oynons and pboyle hem. and mynce hem ſmale and do þ to. colo it with blode and do þ to powdō fort and ſalt and boyle it wele and ſūe it fort ᶠ.

## Roo ᵍ broth. XIIII.

Take the lire of the Deer oþ of the Roo pboile it on ſmale peces ſeeþ it wel half in wat and half in wyne. take brede and bray it wiþ the ſelf broth and drawe blode þ to and lat it feeth to gedre w powdō fort of gyng oþ of caneñ ᵇ. and macys ⁱ. with a grete porcion of vineḡ with Rayſons of Corānte ᵏ.

ᵈ oþ Other, i. e. or
ᵉ temp it. Temper it, i. e. mix it.
ᶠ fort Miſwritten for *forth* So again N° 21. 127.
ᵍ Roo Roe The Recipe in MſE¹ N° 5, is very different.
ᵇ Caneñ. Cinnamon
ⁱ macys. Mace V. Preface and Gloſſ.
ᵏ Rayſons or Corānte. Currants. V. Gloſſ.

Tredure.

Tredure[1].  XV.

Take Brede and grate it. make a lyre[m] of rawe ayreñ and do þto Safroñ and powdõ douce. and lye it up[n] w[t] gode broth. and make it as a Cawdel. and do þto a lytel v̄ions.

Monchelet[o].  XVI.

Take Veel oþ Moton and smite it to gobett seeþ it ĩ gode broth. cast þto erbes yhewe[p] gode wyne. and a qñtite of Oynõns mynced. Powdõ fort and Safroñ. and alye it w[t] ayreñ and v̄ions. but lat not seeþ aft̃.

Bukkenade[q].  XVII.

Take Henn[r] oþ Conyng[s] oþ Veel oþ oþ Flesh ā hewe hem to gobett waische it and hit well[t]. grynde

---

[1] Tredure. A Cawdle, but quære the etymon. The French *tres dure* does not seem to answer.

[m] lyre. Mixture.

[n] lye it up. Mix it.

[o] Monchelet. *Monchelet*, Contents.

[p] y hewe. Shred.

[q] Bukkenade. Vide N° 118. qu.

[r] Hennes, including, I suppose, chicken and pullets.

[s] Conynges. Coneys, Rabbits.

[t] hit well. This makes no sense, unless *hit* signifies smite or beat.

C  Almand

[ 18 ]

Almand unblanched. and drawe hem up w̄ þ broth caſt ꝑ inne rayſons of Corance. ſug. Powdō gyng erbes yſtewed in grees [a]. Oynōns and Salt. If it is to to [x] thynne alye it up w̄ flo of ryſe oꝑ with oꝑ thyng and colō it with Safron.

### Connat [c]. XVIII.

Take Connes and pare hē. pyke out the beſt and do hem in a pot of erthe. do þto whyte grece þ he ſtewe þ inne. and lye hem up with hony clarified and with rawe zolk [z] and with a lytell almand mylke and dꝏ þinne powdō fort and Safron. and loke þat it be yleeſſhed [a].

### Drepee [b]. XIX.

Take blanched Almand grynde hem and temp hē up with gode broth take Oynōns a grete qnnte pboyle hē and frye hē and do þto take ſmale brydd [c] pboyle hē and do þto Pellydore [d] and ſalt. and a lytel grece.

[a] Grees Fr., lard, graſſe. N° 19

[x] to to So agair, N° 124. To is tee, v. Gloſſ And too is founrd coup'ed in this manner in *Mirrour for Magiſtrates*, p. 277. 571, and other aauthors

[c] Connat ſeems to be a kind of marmalade of connes, or quinces, from Fr Coing Chaucer, v Coines. Written qnces N° 30.

[z] Yokes, i e of Egge.

[a] yleeſſhed. V. Gloſſ [b] Drepee. Qu.

[c] Oyſdes Piros *Per n taiLſin, o. R. in Indice.*

[d] Pellycore Perhaps *pruitory. Peletour*, 104.

Maw-

Mawmenee ᵉ.                    XX.

Take a pottel of wyne greke. and ii. poñde of fuğ take and clarifye the fuğ with a q̃ntite of wyne ā drawe it thurgh a ſtỹnő in to a pot of erthe take flő of Caneli ᶠ. and medle ᵍ with sū of the wyne ā caſt to gydre. take pyñ ʰ with Dꝗt and frye hē a litell ī grece oꝑ in oyle and caſt hē to gydre. take clowes ⁱ ā flő of cancl hool ᵏ and caſt ꝑto. take powdő gyng. canel. clow. colő it with sāndres a lytel yf hit be nede caſt falt ꝑto. and lat it feeþ warly ˡ with a flowe fyre and not to thyk ᵐ, take brawn ⁿ of Capoñs yteyſed ᵒ. oꝑ of Fesānt teyſed ſmall and caſt ꝑto.

ᵉ Vide Nº 194, where it is called *Mawmenny*.

ᶠ Flour of Canell. Powder of Cinamon.

ᵍ medle. Mix

ʰ pynes. A nut, or fruit. Vide Gloſſ.

ⁱ clowes. Cloves.

ᵏ hool. Whole. How can it be the flour, or powder, if whole? Quære, *flower* of cand for *mace*.

ˡ warly. Warily, gently.

ᵐ not to thyk. So as to be too thick, or perhaps, *not to thicken.*

ⁿ brawn. Fleſhy part. Few Capons are cut now except about Darking in Surry, they have been excluded by the turkey, a more magnificent, but perhaps not a better fowl.

ᵒ yteyſed, or *teyſed*, as afterwards. Pulled in pieces by the fingers called *teezing* Nº 36. This is done now with fleſh of turkeys, and thought better than mincing. Vide Junius, voce *Teaſe*.

Egurdouce ᵖ. XXI.

Take Conyng or Kydde and ſmyte hem on pecys rawe. and frye hem in white grece. take rayſons of Corance and fry hē take oynons pboile hem and hewe hem ſmall and fry hem. take rede wyne ſug wt powdo of pep. of gyng of canel. ſalt. and caſt þto. and lat it feeþ with a gode qntite of white grece ā ſue it forth.

Capons in Concy ᵠ. XXII.

Take Capons and roſt hem right hoot þat þey be not half y nouhȝ and hewe hem to gobett and caſt hem ī a pot, do þto clene broth, ſeeþ hem þ þey be tendre. take brede and þ ſelf broth and drawe it up yfer ʳ, take ſtrong Powdo and Safron and Salt and caſt þto. take ayren and ſeeþ hem harde. take out the zolk and hewe the whyte þinne, take the Pot fro þ fyre and caſt the whyte þinne. meſſe the diſsh þwith and lay the zolkes hool and flo it with clow.

---

ᵖ Egurdouce. The term expreſſes *piccante dolce*, a mixture of ſour and ſweet, but there is nothing of the former in the compoſition. Vide Gloſſ.

ᵠ Concys ſeems to be a kind of known ſauce. V. Gloſſ.

ʳ yfere. Togethᵉ.

[ 21 ]

### Hares [s] in Talbotes [t]. XXIII.

Take Hares and hewe hem to gobett and seeþ hẽ wt þe blode unwaifshed in broth. and whan þey buth y nouh. caft hem in colde wa͞t. pyke and waifshe hẽ clene. cole [u] the broth and drawe it thuigh a ftynõ, take oþ blode and caft in boylyng wa͞t feeþ it and drawe it thurgh a ftynõ. take Almãnd unblanched. waifshe hem and grynde hem and temp it up with the felf broth. caft al in a pot. tak oynõns and pboile hẽ fmyte hem fmall and caft hem in to þis Pot. caft þinne Powdõ fort. vyneg ã falt.

### Hares in Papdele [x]. XXIIII.

Take Hares pboile hem in gode broth. cole the broth and waifshe the fleyfsh. caft azeyn [y] to gydre. take obleys [z] oþ wafrõus [a] in ftede of lozeyns [b]. and cowche [c] in dyfshes. take powdõ douce and lay on falt the bro͞th and lay onoward [d] ã meffe forth.

---

[s] Haares, Contents. So again, N° 24.
[t] Talbotes. Mf. Ed. N° 9, *Talbotays*.
[u] Cole. Cool.    [x] Papdele Qu.    [y] azeyn. Again.
[z] obleys, called *oblatæ*, for which fee Hearne ad Lib Nig I. p. 344 A kind of Wafer, otherwife called *Nebulæ*, and is the French *oublie*, *oble*. Leland, Collect. IV. p. 190 327.
[a] wafrõns. Wafers.      [b] lofeyns. Vide Gloff.
[c] cowche Lay.
[d] onoward. Upon it

Connyng

Connyng in Cynee ᶜ     xxv.

Take Coñyng and ſmyte hem on peces. and ſecþ hem in gode broth. mynce Oynoñs and ſeeþ hē in grece and in gode broth do þto. drawe a lyre of brede. blode. vyneg and broth do þto with powdo fort.

Connyng in Grauey.     xxvi.

Take Cōnyng ſmyte hem to pecys. þboile hem and drawe hem with a gode broth with almand blanched and brayed. do þinne ſug and powdo gyng and boyle it and the fleſh þwith. flo it w̃ ſug ā w̃ powdo gyng ā ſūeþ forth.

Chykens in Gravey.     xxvii.

Take Chykens and ſūe in the ſame mañe and ſūe forth.

Fylett ᶠ of Galyntyne ᵍ.     xxviii.

Take fylett of Pork and roſt hem half ynowh ſmyte hem on pecys. drawe a lyõ of brede and blode. and broth and Vineg. and do þinne. ſeeþ it wele. and do þinne powdo ā ſalt ā meſſe it forth.

ᶜ Cynee. Vide Gloſſ     ᶠ Fylettes. Fillets.
ᵍ of Galyntyne  In Galyntyne. Contents, red is  As for Ga
lrttre, ſee the Gloſſ.

[ 23 ]

#### Pygg̅ in ſawſe Sawge ʰ.  XXIX.

Take Pigg̅ yſkaldıd and quart he͞ and ſeeþ hem in wat̅ and ſalt, take hem and lat hem keleⁱ. take pſel ſawge. and grynde it with brede and zolkes of ayren͞ harde yſode. temp it up with vyneg̅ ſu͞ what thyk. and lay the Pygg̅ in a veſſell. and the ſewe onoward and ſu͞e it forth.

#### Sawſe madame.  XXX.

Take ſawge. pſel. yſope. and ſau̅ay. qnces. and peer̅ ʰ, garlek and Grapes. and fylle the gees þerwith. and ſowe the hole þat no grece come out. and rooſt hem wel. and kepe the grec̅e þ fallith þof. take galyntyne and grece and do in a poſſynet, whan the gees buth roſted ynouh' take a͞ ſmyte hem on pecys. and þat tatˡ is withinne and do it in a poſſynet and put þinne wyne if it be to thyk. do þto powdo̅ of galyngale. powdo̅ douce and ſalt and boyle the ſawſe and dreſſe þ Gees ī diſhes a͞ lay þ ſowe onoward.

---

ʰ Sawge. Sage. As ſeveral of them are to be uſed, theſe pigs muſt have been ſmall.

ⁱ kele. Cool.

ᵏ Peares. Pears.

ˡ that tat, i. e. that that. Vide Gloſſ.

Gees

### Gees in hoggepot ᵐ. XXXI.

Take Gees and ſmyte hem on pecys. caſt hem in a Pot do þ̉to half wyne and half waƚ. and do þ̉to a gode qn̄tite of Oɉnōs and erbesƚ. Set it oūeʳ it faſt. make a laẏo of brede and blode ā lay it þ̉with. do þ̉to powd̉o fort and sūe it forƚ.

### Carnel ᵒ of Pork. XXXII.

Take the braw̄n of Swyne. pboile it and grynde it ſmale and alay it up with zolkes of ayren. ſet it oūeᵖ the fyre with white Grece and lat it not ſeeþ to faſt. do þ̉inne Safron̄ ā powd̉o fort and meſſe it forth. and caſt þ̉inne powd̉o douce. and sūe it forth.

### Chyken̄s ᵍ in Cawdel. XXXIII.

Take Chiken̄s and boile hem in gode broth and ramm̆eʳ hem up. þenne take zolk̉ of ayren ā þe broth and alɉe it togedre. do þ̉to powd̉o of gyng̉ and ſug̉ ynowh ſafron̄ and ſalt. and ſet it oūe the fyre withoute boyllyng. and sūe the Chɉken̄s holeˢ oþ̉ ybroke and lay þ̇ ſowe onoward.

---

ᵐ Hoggepot. Hodge-podge. *Ochepot.* Mſ. Ed. Nᵒ 22 French, *Hoch-pot* Cotgrave. See Junii Etym v *Hotch-potch.*

ⁿ coūe. Cover     ᵒ Carnel, perhaps *Charnel*, from Fr. *Chaire.*

ᵖ oūe. Over. So again, Nᵒ 33

ᵍ Chɉkens Contents. So again in the next Recipe.

ʳ ramme. Qu preſs them cloſe together.     ˢ hole. Whole.

**Chykens**

Chykens in hocchee [t].                XXXIIII.

Take Chykens and fcald hem. take pſel and fawge withoute eny oþe erbes. take garlec ā grap and ſtoppe the Chikens ful and feeþ hem in gode broth. ſo þat þey may efely be boyled þinne. meſſe hē ā caſt þto powdo dowce.

For to boile Fefant. Ptruch. Capons and Curlew.
                                         XXXV.

Take gode broth and do þto the Fowle. and do þto hool pep and flo of canel a gode qntite and lat hem feeþ þwith. and meſſe it forth. and þ caſt þon Podo dowce.

Blank Mãng [u].                XXXVI.

Take Capons and feeþ hem, þenne take hem up. take Almand blanched. grynd hē and alay hē up with the fame broth caſt the mylk in a pot. waiſhe rys and do þto and lat it feeþ. þanne take brawn of Capons teere it ſmall and do þto. take white grece fug and falt and caſt þinne. lat it feeþ. þenne meſſe it

---

[t] Hochee. This does not at all anſwer to the French *Hachis*, or our *Haſh*, therefore qu

[u] Blank Mãng. Very different from ours. Vide Gloſſ.

forth and florish it with aneys in confyt rede oþ whyt. and with Almaṇd fryed in oyle. and sūe it forth.

### Blank Defforre [z]. XXXVII.

Take Almaṇd blanched, grynde hem and temp hem up with whyte wyne, on fleifsh day with broth. and cast þinne flo of Rys. oþ amydōn [y], and lye it þwith. take brawn of Capons ygroñd. take fug and falt and cast j to and florish it with aneys whyte. take a veffel yholes [z] and put in fafron. and sūe it forth.

### Morree [a]. XXXVIII.

Take Almand blanched. waifshe hem. grynde hem. and temp hem up with rede wyne, and alye hem wt flo of Rys. do j to Pyn j fryed. and coloꝛ it with sandi. do þto powdoꝛ fort and powdoꝛ douce and falt. meffe it forth and flo it [b] with aneys confyt whyte.

---

[z] Blank Defforre. V. Gl ff.

[y] Amydon. "Fine wheat flour fleeped in water, ftrained and let ftand to fettle, then made a red and dried in the fun, ufed for bread or in broths." Cotgrave. Ufed in Nº 68 for colouring white.

[z] yholes. Quære

[a] Morree. Ms. Ed. 37 morry. Ibid II 26, morrey, probably from its mulberry colour therein.

[b] flo. Equal it.

Charlet.

### Charlet [c]. XXXIX.

Take Pork and feeþ it wel. hewe it fmale. caſt it in a panne. breke ayren̄ and do þto and fwyng [d] it wel togyder. do þto Cowe mylke and Safron̄ and boile it togȳd. falt it & meſſe it forth.

### Charlet yforced. XXII.

Take mylke and feeþ it, and fwyng þwith zolkes of Ayren̄ and do þto. and powdo of gyng ſug. and Safron̄ and caſt þto. take the Charlet out of the broth and meſſe it ī dyſshes, lay the fewe onoward. flo it with powdo douce. and sūe it forth.

### Cawdel ferry [e]. XXII. I.

Take flo of Payndemayn [f] and gode wyne. and drawe it togydre. do þto a grete q̄ntite of Sug cypre. or hony clarified. and do þto ſafron̄. boile it. and whan it is boiled, alye it up with zolkes of ayren̄. and do þto ſalt and meſſe it forth. and lay þon ſug and powdo gyng.

---

[c] Charlet, probably from the French, *chair*. Qu. Minced Meat, and the next article, Forced Meat

[d] fwyng. Shake, mix.

[e] ferry. Quære We have *Carpe in Ferry*, Lel. Coll. VI. p. 21.

[f] Payndemayn. White bread. Chaucer.

Jusshell [g].     XX II. III.

Take brede ygrated and ayren and swyng it to-gydre. do þto safron, sawge. and salt. ⁊ cast broth. þto. boile it & messe it forth.

Jusshell enforced [h].     XX II. IIII.

Take and do þto as to charlet yforced. and sue it forth.

Mortrews [i].     XX II. V.

Take henn and Pork and seeþ hem togyd. take the lyre of Henn and of the Pork, and hewe it small and gnde it all to doust [k]. take brede ygted and do þto, and temp it with the self broth and alye it with zolk of ayren, and cast þon powdo fort, boile it and

---

[g] Jusshell See also next number *J. sell*, Mr Ed 21, where the Recipe is much the same Lat *Juscell* which occurs in the ch Chorast on Juvenal n 23, a — 11 Apicius, v 3 V de Du Fresne, v *Ju ellum* and *Jus* ' -, where the composition consists of - rum, ova, and /13 ... very different from this Laber in Thesauro *e Ju e* —, *æ* from 'L cod P iscinus

N. B. N° XX. II. is omitted both here and in the Contents.

[h] Jusnell enforced As the *Charlet yforced* here referred to was made of pork, compare N° 40 with N° 39 So in Theod. Priscian we have *Jusse L in Gallinæ*

[i] Mortrews Vide Goff.

[k] doust. Dust, powder.

to

do þin powdʳ of gyngᵈ fugᵈ. fafron and falt. and loke
þ it be ftondyng¹, and flo it with powdʳ gyng.

### Mortrews blank.  XX II. VI.

Take Pork and Henn and feeþ hem as to fore. bray
almand blanched, and temp hem up with the felf broth.
and alye the fleifsh with the mylke and white flo of
Rys. and boile it. & do þin powdʳ of gyngᵈ fugar and
look þat it be ftondyng.

### Brewet of Almony ᵐ.  XX II. VII.

Take Conyng or kidd and hewe hem fmall on
mofcels ⁿ oþ on pecys. þboile hem w ͭ the fame broth,
drawe an almande mylke and do the fleifsh þwith, caft
þto powdʳ galyngale & of gyng with flo of Rys. and
colʳ it wiþ alkenet. boile it, falt it. & meffe it forth
with fugᵈ and powdʳ douce.

### Peions ᵒ yftewed.  XX II. VIII.

Take peions and ftop hem with garlec ypylled and
with gode erbes ihewe. and do hem in an erthen pot.

---

¹ ftondyng. Stiff, thick.

ᵐ Almony. Almaine, or Germany *Almany*. Fox, part I p.
239. *Alamanie* Chron Sax p 242. V. ad Nᵒ 71.

ⁿ mofcels Morfels

ᵒ Peions, Pejons, i. e. Pigeons. ȝ is never written here in the
middle of a word.

caft

caſt þto gode broth and whyte grece. Powdõ fort.
saffroñ vions & ſalt.

## Loſeyns P.   XXII. IX.

Take gode broth and do ī an erthen pot, take flõ
of payndemayn and make þ of paſt with waɫ. and make
þof thynne foyles as p-p ꝗ with a roller, drye it harde
and ſeeþ it ī broth take Cheſe ruayn ʳ grated and lay
it in difsh with powdõ douce. and lay þon loſeyns
iſode as hoole as þou mızt ˢ and above powdõ and
cheſe, and ſo twyſe or thryſe, & sũe it forth.

## Tarleti ᵗ.   XXII. X.

Take pork yſode and grynde it ſmall with ſaffroñ,
medle it with ayreñ and raiſons of corounce and powdõ fort and ſalt. and make a foile of dowhȝ ᵘ and
cloſe the fars ˣ þinne. caſt þ Tartlet ī a Panne with
faire waɫ boillyng and ſalt, take of the clene Fleſsh
withoute ayreñ ꝫ boile it ī gode broth. caſt þto powdõ

---

ᵖ Loſeyns. Vide in Gloſſ.

ꝗ foyles as pap. Leaves of paſte as thin as paper.

ʳ Cheſe ruyan   166. Vide Gloſſ

ˢ mızt. Might, i e can

ᵗ Tarlettes. Tartletes, in the proceſs.

ᵘ foile of dowhz, or dowght. A leaf of paſte

ˣ fars. Forced-meat.

douce

douce and ſalt, and meſſe the tartletꝭ in diſſhꝭ & heldeʸ the ſewe jꝯonne.

### Pynnonade ᶻ. XX. II XI.

Take Almandꝭ iblãched and drawe hem ſũdell thicke ᵃ with gode broth oꝑ with waꝼ and ſet on the fire and ſeeþ it, caſt ꝑto zolkꝭ of ayren̄ ydrawe. take Pyn̄ yfꝛyed in oyle oꝑer in grece and ꝑto white Powdoꝛ douce, ſugꝛ and ſalt. & coloꝛ it wiþ alkenet a lytel.

### Roſee ᵇ. XX. II. XII.

Take thyk mylke as to foꝛe welled ᶜ. caſt ꝑto ſugꝛ a gode porciõn pyn̄. Dates ymynced. canel. & powdoꝛ gyng and ſeeþ it, and alye it with flõs of white Roſis, and flõꝛ of ꝛys, cole it, ſalt it & meſſe it forth. If þ wilt in ſtede of Almãde mylke, take ſwete crem̄ of kyne.

### Cormarye ᵈ. XX. II. XIII.

Take Colyandꝛe ᵉ, Caraway ſmale groñden, Powdoꝛ of Pep and garlec ygroñde in ꝛede wyne, medle alle

---
ʸ helde. Caſt.

ᶻ *Pynnonade*   So named from the *Pynes* therein uſed.

ᵃ ſũdell thicke   Somewhat thick, thickiſh

ᵇ *Roſee*   From the white roſes therein mentioned. See Nº 41. in MS. Ed. but Nº 47 there is totally different

ᶜ welled, f. as *l'ed*, directed.

ᵈ Cormarye. Quære.     ᵉ Colyandre. Coriander.

[ 32 ]

ꝼiſe [f] togyd and ſalt it, take loyn of Pork rawe and fle of the ſwyn. and pryk it wel with a knyf and lay it in the ſawſe, rooſt þof what þ wilt, & kepe þat þ falluth ꝼfro ĩ the roſting and ſeeþ it in a poſſynet with faire broth, & ſerue it forth wiþ þ rooſt anoon [g].

### Newe Noumbles of Deer. II. XXIIII.

Take noumbles and waiſshe hem clene with waꝛ and ſalt and pboile hē ĩ waꝛ. take hē up ã dyce hē. do w hē as w ooþ noumbles.

### Nota. II. XXV.

The Loyne of the Pork, is fro the hippe boon to the hede.

### Nota. II. XXVI.

The fylet buth two, that buth take oute of the Peſtels [i].

### Spynee [k]. II. XXVII.

Take and make gode thik Almãnd mylke as tofore. and do þin of fio of hawtherñ [l]. and make it as a roſe. & ſerue it forth.

---

[f] þiſe Theſe       [g] anoon. Immediately.
[i] Peſtels Legs
[k] Spynee As made of Haws, the berries of Spires, or Hawthorrs.
[l] Hawtherñ. Hawthorn.

Chyryſe.

[ 33 ]

### Chyryſe¹.   *xk.* II. XVIII.

Take Almãd unblanched, waiſhe hem, grynde hem, drawe hem up with godė broth. do þto thridde part of chiryſe. þ ſtoñ. take oute and grynde hem ſmale, make a layõ of gode brede ā powdõ and ſalt and do þto. colõ it with ſandr̃ ſo that it may be ſtondyng, and floriſh it with aneys and with cheweryes, and ſtrawe þuppon and ſũe it forth.

### Payn Fondewᵐ.   *xx* II. XIX.

-Take brede and frye it iñ grece oþ in oyle, take it and lay it in rede wyne. grynde it w̃ raiſons take hony and do it in a pot and caſt þinne gleyrⁿ of ayrẽ wiþ a litel wat̃ and betė it wele togider with a ſklyſeᵒ. ſet it oũe the fir̃ and boile it. and whan the hatteᵖ ariſith to goonᑫ oũe. take it adõn and kele it, and whan it is þ clarifiedr̃ do it to the oȝe with ſug̃ and ſpices.

---

¹ Chyryſe. *Chiryſ.* in the proceſs. *Cheriſye.* Mſ Ed. II. 18 *Chiryes* there are cherries And this diſh is evidently made of Cherries, which probably were chiefly imported at this time from Flanders, though they have a Saxon name, cyrṛe.

ᵐ fõndewe. Contents. It ſeems to mean *diſſolved.* V. *fornd* in Glſſ.

ⁿ glevres. Whites.      ᵒ Sklyſe Slice.

ᵖ hatte. Seems to mean *bubling* or *v allop.*

ᑫ goon. Go.

E                                         ſalt

falt it and loke it be ftondyng, florifh it with white coliandre in confyt.

### Croton ⁿ.                                          XX. III.

Take the offal of Capons oþ of oþe bridd. make hē clene and pboile hem. take hem up and dyce hem. take fwete cowe mylke and caft þinne. and lat it boile. take Payndemayn ⁿ and of þ felf mylke and drawe thurgh a cloth and caft it in a pot and lat it feeþ. take ayren yfode. hewe the white and caft þto. and alye the fewe with zolkes of ayren rawe. colo it with fafron. take the zolkes and fry hem and florifh hem þwith and with powdo douce.

### Vyne grace ⁿ.                                      XX. III. I.

Take fmale fylett of Pork and roft hem half and fmyte hem to gobett and do hem in wyne ā Vyneg and Oynons; mynced and ftewe it yfere do þto. gode powdos ā falt. ā sue it forth.

---

ⁿ Croton. Mſ Ed 24 has Craytōa, but a different difh.

ⁿ Payndemayn. Whitebread. V. ad Nº 41.

ⁿ Vyne Grace. Named probably from gras, wild fwine, and the mode of creſſing in ſ" ie. V. Gloſſ voce ſj e g acc

Fohnell.

[ 35 ]

### Fonnell ᵘ.     XX III. II.

Take Almand unblanched. grynde hem and drawe hem up with gode broth. take a lombe ˣ or a kidde and half roſt hȳ. or the þridde ʸ part, ſmyte hym ī gobet and caſt hym to the mylke. take ſmale bridd yfaſted and yſtyned ᶻ. and do þto ſug, powdo of canell and ſalt, take ʒolkes of ayren harde yſode and cleene ᵃ a two and ypanced ᵇ with flo of canell and floriſh þ ſewe above. take alkenet fryed and yfondred ᶜ and droppe above with a feþ ᵈ and meſſe it forth.

### Douce ame ᵉ.     XX III. III.

Take gode Cowe mylke and do it in a pot. take pſel. ſawge. yſope. ſauay and ooþ gode herbes. hewe hem and do hem in the mylke and ſeeþ hem. take capons half yroſted and ſmyte hem on pecys and do þto pyn and hony clarified. ſalt it and colo it with ſafron ā ſue it forth.

---

ᵘ Fonnell. Nothing in the recipe leads to the etymon of this multifarious diſh.

ˣ Lombe. Lamb.     ʸ thridde. Third, per metatheſin.
ᶻ yfaſted and yſtyned.     ᵃ cleeue. cloven.
ᵇ ypanced. pounced.     ᶜ yfondred. melted, diſſolved.
ᵈ feþ'. feather.

ᵉ Douce Ame. *Quaſi*, a delicious diſh. V. Blank Deſire in Gloſſ. Titles of this tiſſue occur in Apicius. See Humelberg. p. 2

[ 36 ]

### Connyng in Cyrip f.    III. IIII.

Take Conyng and seeþ hem wel i good broth. take wyne greke and do þto with a porcion of vyneg and flo of canel, hoole clow quybibes hoole. and ooþ gode spices with raisons coraunce and gyngyn ypared and ymynced. take up the conyng and smyte hem on pecys and cast hem into the Siryppe and seeþ hem a litel on the fyr and sue it forth.

### Leche Lumbard g.    III. V.

Take rawe Pork and pulle of the skyn and pyke out þ skyn synew and bray the Pork in a mort w ayren rawe do þto sug, salt, raysons corance, dat mynced, and powdo of Pep powdo gylofre. a do it i a bladder, and lat it seeþ til it be ynowh3. and whan it is ynowh, kerf it lesshe it h in likenesse of a peskodde i, and take grete raysons and grynde hem in a mort, drawe hem up wiþ rede wyne, do þto mylke of almand colo it with sanders a safron. and do þto powdo of pep a of

---

f Cyrip  In the procefs Siryppe  Cirypp, Contents. Sirop, or Sirup, as 133. Syryp, 132.

g Leche Lumbard. So called from the country. Randle Home fays Leach is "a kind of jelly made of cream, ising-glafs, sugar "and almonds, with other compounds."

h Leshe it. Vide Gloff

i Pefkodde. Hull or pod of a pea

gilofre

gilofre and boile it. and whan it is iboiled take powdͬ
of canel and gynḡ, and tēp it up with wyne. and do
alle þiſe thyng togȳd. and loke þat it be rēnyns ᵏ, and
lat it not seeþ aft that it is caſt togyder, ā sūe it
forth,

### Connyng in clere broth.     XV. III. VI.

Take Coñyng and ſmyte hem ĩ gobet and waiſsh
hem and do hem in feyre waͨ and wyne, and seeþ
hem and ſkym hem. and whan þey buth iſode pyke
hem clene, and drawe the broth thurgh a ſtȳnͦ and
do the fleſsh þwith ĩ a Poſſynet and ſtyne it ˡ. and do
þto vyneǵ and powdͦ of gyng and a grete q̃ntite and
ſalt aft the laſt boillyng and sūe it forth,

### Payn Ragoñ ᵐ.     XX. III. VII.

Take hony ſug and clariſie it togydre. and boile
it with eſy fȳr, and kepe it wel fͦ brēnyng and whan
it hath yboiled a while; take up a drope ⁿ þof wiþ þy
fyng̃ and do it in a litel waͨ and loke if it hong ͦ togyder, and take it fro the fyre and do þto the thrid-

---

ᵏ rēnyns. Perhaps *thin*, from the old *renne*, to run. Vide Gloſſ.
ˡ ſtyne it. Cloſe it. V. Gloſſ.
ᵐ Payn ragōn It is not at all explained in the Recipe,
ⁿ Drope Drop.
ᵒ hong. Hing, or hang.

-dendele

-dendele ᵖ ã powdͦ gyngeñ and stere ᵠ it togyd til it bi-
gynne to thik and cast it on a wete ʳ table. lesh it
and sue it forth w̃ fryed mete on flesh day oɪ on
fyshe dayes.

Lete Lardes ˢ.                     III. VIII.

Take psel and grynde with a Cowe mylk, medle it
with ayreñ and lard ydyced take mylke aft þ þ hast
to done ᵗ and myng ᵘ þwith. and make ʃof dyuse colours. If þ wolt have zelow, do þto safroñ and no
psel. If þ wolt have it white, nonþ psel ne safroñ
but do þto amydoñ. If þ wilt have rede do þto san-
dres. If þou wilt have pownas ˣ do þto turnesole ʸ.
If þ wilt have blak do þto blode ysode and fryed. and
set on the f,r̄ i as many vessels as þ hast colours þerto

ᵖ thriddendele. Third part, perhaps, *of brede*, i. e. of bread,
may be casually omitted here. V Gloss

ᵠ stere. stir.                     ʳ wete. wet.

ˢ Lete Lardes. *Lard,* in form of Dice are noticed in the process.
See Lel Coll. VI p. 5. *Lete* is the Fr *Lait*, milk. V Nº 81.
or Brit. *Llaeth* Hence, perhaps, *Lethe Cyprus* and *Lethe Rubi*.
Leˡ Coll IV p 227. But VI. p. 5, it is *Leche*.

ᵗ to done, i e. done.

ᵘ myng. mix.

ˣ pownas. Qu.

ʸ turnesole. Not the flower *Heliotrope*, but a drug. Northumb.
Book, p. 3. 19. I suppose it to be *Turmeric* V. Brooke's Nat.
Hist. of Vegetables, p. 9 where it is used both in victuals and for
dying.

and

[ 39 ]

and seeþ it wel and lay þise colours i̅ a cloth first oon, and sithen anoþ upon him. and sithen the þridde and the ferthe. and p̅sse it harde til it be all out clene. And whan it is al colde, lesh it thynne, put it i̅ a panne and fry it wel. and su̅e it forth.

### Furmente with Porpays [z].    XV. III. IX.

Take Almand blanched. bray hem and drawe hem up with faire wat̅, make furmente as before [a] and cast þ furmente þto. ⁊ messe it with Porpays.

### Perrey of Peson̅ [b].    XX III. X.

Take peson̅ and seeþ hem fast and cove hem til þei berst. þenne take up hem and cole hem thurgh a cloth. take oynons and mynce he̅ and seeþ hem in the same sewe and oile þwith, cast þto sugur, salt and safron̅, and seeþ hem wel þast and su̅e hem forth.

### Peson of Almayne [c].    XX III. XI.

Take white peson̅, waishe hem seeþ hem a grete while. take hem and cole hem thurgh a cloth, waishe

---

[z] Porpays. *Porpeys*, Contents, and so N° 116. Porpus.

[a] as before. This is the first mention of it

[b] Perrey of Peson̅, i. e. Pens *Perrey* seems to mean pulp; vide N° 73 Mr Ozell in Rabelais, IV. c. 60. renders *Puree de pois* by *Peas soup*.

[c] Almayne Germain, called Almony N° 47.

hem

hem ĩ cōlde wa͞t til the hulles go off, caſt hem in a pot and coūe þ no breth ᵈ go out. and boile hem right wel. and caſt þinne gode mylke of almand and a ptye of flo of Rys wiþ powdͦ gyng ſafron. and ſalt.

### Chych ᵉ.    xx III. XII.

Take chich and wry hem ᶠ ĩ aſhes all nyȝt, oþ lay hem in hoot aymers ᵍ, at morrowe ʰ, waiſhe heᵯ in clene wa͞t and do hem oūe the fire with clene wa͞t. ſeeþ hē up and do þto oyle, garlec, hole ſafroᵯ. powdͦ fort and ſalt, ſeeþ it and meſſe it forth.

### Frenche ⁱ.    xx III. XIII.

Take and ſeeþ white peſon and take oute þ perrey ᵏ ᛬ þboile erbis ᛬ hewe hē grete ᛬ caſt hē ĩ a pot w the perrey pulle oynoᵯs ᛬ ſeeþ hē hole wel ĩ wa͞t ᛬ do hē to þ Perrey w oile ᛬ ſalt, colͦ it w ſafroᵯ ᛬ meſſe it and caſt þon powdͦ douce.

---

ᵈ breth. Breath, air, ſteam. Mſ Ed Nº 2.

ᵉ Chyches. *Viciæ*, vetches. In Fr. *Ch cles*.

ᶠ wry hem. *Dry h-m*, or *cover hom* Chaucer, v. wtey.

ᵍ Aymers. Embers, of which it is evidently a corruption.

ʰ at morrowe. Next Morning.

ⁱ Frenche. Contents have it more fully, *Frenche Owtes*. V. ad Nº 6.

ᵏ Perrey. Pulp V. ad Nº 70.

### Makke¹.           XXIII. XIIII.

Take drawen benes and seeþ hē wel. take hē up of the watˉ and cast hē in a mort grynde hem al to doust til þei be white as eny mylk, chawfᵐ a litell rede wyne, cast þͨamong in þ gryndyng, do þͬto salt, leshe it ī difsh. þanne take Oynoñs and mynce hem smale and seeþ hem ī oile til þey be al broñⁿ. and florish the difsh þͬwithͬ. and sūe it forth.

### Aquapatys°.        XXIII. XV.

Pill garlec and cast it in a pot with watˉ and oile. and seeþ it, do þͬto safroñ, salt, and powdoͬ fort and dresse it forth hool.

### Salat.           XXIII. XVI.

Take psel, sawge, garlec, chiboliͬ, oynoñs, leek, borage, mynt, porrectᵖ, fenel and ton tressisᵠ, rew, rosemarye, purslaryeʳ, laue and waische hem clene,

---

¹ Makke. *Ignotum.*
ᵐ Chawf   Warm.
ⁿ broñ.   Brown.
° Aquapatys. *Aquapates,* Contents. Perhaps named from the water used in it.
ᵖ Porrectes   Fr *Porrette.*
ᵠ Ton tressis   Cresses. V. Gloss.
ʳ Purslarye.   P[urs]lan.

pike hem, pluk hē fmall wiþ þyn ˢ honde and myng hem wel with rawe oile. lay on vyneg and falt, and sūe it forth.

### Fenkel in Soppes.    XX III. XVII.

Take blades of Fenkel. ſhrede hem not to ſmale, do hem to ſeeþ in waꝉ and oile and oynons mynced þwith. do þto ſafron and ſalt and powdo. douce. sūe it forth. take brede ytoſted and lay the ſewe onoward.

### Clat ᵗ.    XX III. XVIII.

Take elena campana and ſeeþ it waꝉ ᵘ. take it up and grynde it wel in a mort. temp it up w̃ᵗ ayren ſafron and ſalt and do it ou the fire and lat it not boile. caſt above powdo douce and sūe it forth.

### Appulmoy ˣ.    XX III. XIX.

Take Apples and ſeeþ hem in waꝉ, drawe hem thurgh a ſtyno. take almande mylke & hony and flo of Rys, ſafron and powdo fort and ſalt. and ſeeþ it ſtondyng ʸ.

---

ˢ þyn thire.      ᵗ Clat. Qd
ᵘ water, r in ſtater, as in Nº 79.
ˣ Appulmo, *Appulmos* MS Ed Nº 17. named from the apples employed. V Nº 149
ʸ ſtondyng. thict

Slete

[ 43 ]

### Slete ᶻ Soppes. XX IIII.

Take white of Lekᵉ and flyt hem, and do hem to feþ ĩ wyne, oile and falt, roft brede and lay in dyfsh and the fewe above and sũe it forth.

### Letelorye ᵃ. XX. IIII. I.

Take Ayrẽn and wryng hem thurgh a ſtỹnoᵈ and do þto cowe mylke with buttĩ and fafrõn and falt and feþ it wel. leſhe it. and loke þat it be ſtondyng. and sũe it forth.

### Sowpᵉ Dorry ᵇ. XX IIII. II.

Take Almãnd brayed, drawe hem up with wyne. boile it, caſt þuppon fafiõn and falt, take brede itoſted in wyne. lay þof a leyne ᶜ and anoþ of þ fewe and alle togydre. floriſh it with fugᵈ powdoᵈ gyngᵈ and sũe it forth.

### Rape ᵈ. XX IIII. III.

Take half fygᵉ and half raifõns pike hem and waiſhe hem in wat ſkalde hem in wyne. bray hem in a morf,

---

ᶻ Slete. flit.

ᵃ Letelorye. The latter part of the compound is unknown, the firſt is Fr. *Lait,* milk. Vide N° 68.

ᵇ Sowpes Dorry. Sops endorfed. V. *Dorry* in Gloſſ.

ᶜ A leyne. a layer.

ᵈ Rape. A diſſyllable, as appears from *Rapey* in the Contents. *Rapy,* Mſ. Ed. N° 49. *Rapee,* ibid II 28.

and drawe hem thurgh a strayno͝ur. cast hem in a pot and þwiþ powdo͝ur of pep and ooþ good powdo͝urs. alay it up with flo͝ur of Rys. and colo͝ur it with saundres. salt it. & messe it forth.

     Sawse Sarzyne<sup>e</sup>.    xx    IIII.IIII.

Take hepp͝es and make hem clene. take Almānd͝es blaunched. frye hem in oile and bray hem in a mort with hepp͝es. drawe it up with rede wyne, and do þin sug͝ur ynowh3 with Powdo͝ur fort. lat it be stondyng, and alay it with flo͝ur of Rys. and colo͝ur it with alkenet and messe it forth. and florish it with Pŏme garnet. If þu wilt in fleshe day keeþ Capons and take the brawn and tese hem smal and do þ͝rto. and make the lico<sup>f</sup> of þis broth.

     Creme of Almānd͝es.    xx    IIII.V.

Take Almānd͝es blaunched, grynde hem and drawe hem up thykke, set hem ouer the fyre & boile hem. set hem adoun and spryng<sup>g</sup> hem with Vyneg͝ur, cast hem abrode uppon a cloth and cast uppon hem sug͝ur. whan it is colde gadre it togydre and leshe it in dysh͝es.

---

<sup>e</sup> Sawse Sarzyne. *Staffs* Contents *Saracer*, we presume, from the nation or people. There is a Recipe in MS Ed. N° 54 for a Bruet of *Sarcynesse*, but there are no pomgranates concerned

<sup>f</sup> Lco. liquor.      <sup>g</sup> spryng. sprinkle.

                Grewel

[ 45 ]

### Grewel of Almand.   XX IIII. VI.

Take Almānd blānched. bray hē w̄ oot meel ʰ, and draw hē up with waī. caſt p̄on Safron ⁊ ſalt ⁊c.

### Cawdel of Almānd mylk.   XX IIII. VII.

Take Almānd blānched and drawe hem up with wyne, do p̄to powdͬ of gyng̃ and ſug̃ and colͬ it with Safron. boile it and ſūe it forth.

### Jowt of Almānd Mylke.   XX IIII. VIII.

Take erbes, boile hem, hewe hem and grynde hem ſmale. and drawe hem up with waī. ſet hem on the fire and ſeeþ the rowt with the mylke. and caſt p̄on ſug̃ ⁊ ſalt. ⁊ ſūe it forth.

### Fygey ᵏ.   XX IIII. IX.

Take Almānd blanched, grynde hem and drawe hem up with waī and wyne · quaīt fyg̃ hole raiſons. caſt p̄to powdͬ gyng̃ and hony clarified. ſeeþ it wel ⁊ ſalt it, and ſūe forth.

---

ʰ oot meel. oat-meal.
ⁱ Jowtes. V. ad N° 60.
ᵏ Fygey. So named from the figs therein uſed. A different Recipe, Mſ. Ed. N° 3, has no figs.

Pochee.

[ 46 ]

#### Pochee¹.   XX IIII. X.

Take Ayren̄ and breke hem ī fcaldyng hoot wat̄. an̄ whan þei bene fode ynowh. take hē up and take zulkes of ayren and rawe mylke and fwyng hem togvdre, and do þto powdo gyng̃ fafron̄ and falt, fet it oūe the fire, and lat it not boile, and take ayren̄ ifode ⁊ caſt þ few onoward. ⁊ sūe it forth.

#### Brewet of Ayrēn.   XX IIII. XI.

Take ayren̄, wat̄ and butt̄, and feeþ hem yfere with fafron̄ and gobett of chefe. wryng ayren̄ thurgh a ſtraynō. whan the wat̄ hath foden awhile, take þēne the ayren̄ and fwyng hē with vious. and caſt þto. fet it oūe the fire and lat it not boile. and sūe it forth.

#### Macrows ᵐ.   XX IIII XII.

Take and make a thynne foyle of dowh. and kerve it on peces, and caſt hem on boillyng wat̄ ⁊ feeþ it wele. take chefe and grate it and butt̄ caſt bynethen and above as lofyns. and sūe forth.

---

¹ Pochee. Poached eggs. Very different from the prefent way.

ᵐ Macrows *Maccherore*, according to the Recipe in *Altieri*, correfponds nearly enough with our procefs, fo that this title feems to want mending, and yet I know not how to do it to fatisfaction.

### Toſtee [n].  XX IIII. XIII.

Take wyne and hony and foñd it [o] togẏd and ſkym it clene. and ſeeþ it long, do ⁹þto powdõ of gynḡ. pep and ſalt, toſt brede and lay the ſew ⁹þto. kerue pecys of gynḡ and flõ it ⁹þwith and meſſe it forth.

### Gyngawdry [p].  XX IIII. XIIII.

Take the Powche [q] and the Lyuõ [r] of haddok, cod-lyng and hake [s] and of ooþ fiſhe, ⁹þboile hē, take hē and dyce hem ſmall, take of the ſelf broth and wyne, a layõ of brede of galyntyne with gode powdõs and ſalt, caſt þat fyſshe ⁹þinne and boile it. ⁊ do ⁹þto amy-doñ. ⁊ colõ it grene.

### Erbowle [t].  XX. IIII. XV.

Take bolas and ſcald hem with wyne and drawe hem with [u] a ſtẏnõ do hem in a pot, clarify hony and do ⁹þto with powdõ fort. and flõ of Rys. Salt it ⁊ floriſh it w[t] whyte aneys. ⁊ sũe it forth.

---

[n] Toſtee. So called from the coaſted bread.
[o] fõnd it. mix it   [p] Gyngawdry. Qu.
[q] Powche. Crop or ſtomach.
[r] Lyuõ. Liver. V. N° 137.
[s] Hake. "Aſellus alter, ſive Merlucius, Aldrov." So Mr. Ray. See Pennant, ⅢI p. 156
[t] Erbowle. Perhaps from the *Bolas*, or Bullace employed.
[u] with, i. e. thurgh or thorough.

Reſmolle.

### Refmolle [x].     IIII. XVI.

Take Almãnd blanched and drawe hem up with waṫ and alye it with flõ of Rys and do p̃to powdõ of gyng fug̃ and falt, and loke it be not ftondyng [y], meffe it and sũe it forth.

### Vyande Cypre [z].     IIII. XVII.

Take oot mele and pike out the fton and grynde hem fmale, and drawe hem thurgh a ſtyñõ. take mede oþ wyne ifonded in fug̃ and do þife þinne. do p̃to powdõ and falt, and alay it with flõ of Rys and do þat it be ftondyng. if thou wilt on flefh day take henn and pork yfode ⁊ grynde hem fmale and do p̃to. ⁊ meffe it forth.

### Vyande Cypre of Samoñ [a].     IIII. XVIII.

Take Almaṅd and bray hem unblanched. take cal-

---

[x] Refmlle From the Rice there ufed, for Mf Ed. II. N° 5. has R, f -l, where n y e feems to be Fr moll, as written alfo in the Roll Rice molns porage Lel Coll. VI. p 26

[y] Not ſtondyng Thin, diluted V N° 98 Not to [too] ſtondyng, 121.

[z] Cypre Cpre, Contents here and N° 98.

[a] Samon S. mon.

war

[ 49 ]

war [b] Samõn and seeþ it in lewe watᵉ drawe up þyn almãd with the bioth. pyke out the bon̄ out of the fyſsh clene ⁊ grynde it ſmall ⁊ caſt þy mylk ⁊ þ togẏd ⁊ alye it w̃ flõ of Rys, do þto powdõ fort, ſug̃ ⁊ ſalt ⁊ colõ it w̃ alkenet ⁊ loke þ hit be not ſtondyng and meſſe it forth.

Vyannd Ryal.     IIII. XIX.

Take wyne greke, oþ rynyſshe wyne and hony clarified þwith. take flõ of rys powdõ of Gyng̃ oþ of pep ⁊ canel. oþ flõ of canel. powdõ of clow. ſafron̄. ſug̃ cypre. mylþeiyes, oþ ſañdr. ⁊ medle alle þiſe togid. boile it and ſalt it. and loke þat it be ſtondyng.

Compoſt [d].     c.

Take rote of pſel. paſternak of raſens [e]. ſcrape hem and waiſthe hē clene. take rap ⁊ caboch ypared and

---

[b] calwar Salwar, Nº 167. R. Holme ſays, "*Calver* is a term "uſed to a Flounder when to be boiled in oil, vinegar, and ſpices "and to be kept in it." But in Lancaſhire Salmon newly taken and immediately dreſſed is called *Calver Salmon* and in Littleton *Salar* is a young ſalmon.

[c] lewe water warm V Gloſſ.

[d] Compoſt. A compoſition to be always ready at hand. Holme, III p. 78. Lel. Coll. VI. p 5.

[e] Paſternak of raſēns. Qu.

G     icorne.

[ 50 ]

icorne ᶠ. take an erthen pane wᵗ clene watᵉ ⁊ set it on the fre. cast all þise ꝑinne. whan þey buth boiled cast þto peer ⁊ pboile hem wel take þise thyng up ⁊ lat it kele on a fair c'oth, do ꝛto salt whan it is colde in a vessel take vineg ⁊ powdoᵘ ⁊ safron ⁊ do þto. ⁊ lat alle þise thing l̄ye ꝑin al nyzt oꝛ al day, take wyne greke and hony clarified togȳd lumbarde muſtard ⁊ raisons corance al hool ⁊ grynde powdoᵘ of canel powdoᵘ douce ⁊ aneys hole. ⁊ fenell seed. take alle þise thyng ⁊ cast togȳd ī a pot of erthe. and take þof whan þᵘ wilt ⁊ sue forth.

Geleᵉ of Fyſsh.     c. 1.

Take Tench, pykes ʰ, eelys, turbut and plays ⁱ, kerue hē to pecys. scalde hē ⁊ waiſche hē clene. drye

---

ᶠ ypꝛred and icorne The fi ſt ꝛeꝛates t the Rapes, the second to the Capocheꝛ, and me s c ꝛ c  ꝛn pieces

ᵍ Ge ] ꝛ G⸌, Co ers ere ꝛnd ꝛ the next Recipe. Cꝛ, Mꝛ Eᵈ N° 55, v ꝛ cꝛ pꝛeꝛeꝛs ds ꝛith much the ſame pieſcꝛ ꝛ uꝛ

ʰ It ꝛs commonly thought this fiſh was not e nt in Eng'a d till the re 5 a cꝛ H. VIII , but ſee N° ꝛ07 to ꝛ 114. So Lucys, oꝛ Ten_uꝛ Ml Eᵈ II 1 ꝛ Pygus or Tenchꝛs, II. 2   Pꝑys, 33 Chaucer, ꝛ Luce and Leꝛ Coꝛ IV. p 226. VI p 1 5 Luce ſaꝛ Ibid p 6. Mꝛ Topham's Mſ written about 1250, menꝛions Lꝛpꝛs aqꝛꝛt cos five Lꝛceos ꝛmorgꝛ the fiſh whꝛch the fiſhmonger ꝛ ꝛs to haꝛe in hꝛs ꝛhop   They were the arms of the Lucꝛ ꝛamꝛly ꝛo earlꝛ ꝛs Eꝛw I   See ꝛ fo Pennant's Zool. III. p 280, 4to.

ⁱ Plays. Pꝛaiſꝛ, the fiſh.

hē

hē w̄ a cloth do hē ī a pāne do p̄to half vyneg̃ ꝫ half wvne ꝫ feeþ it wel. ꝫ take the Fyſshe and pike it clene, cole the broth thurgh a cloth īto an erthen pāne. do p̄to powdō of pep̄ and ſafron ynowh. lat it feeþ and ſkym it wel whan it is yſode dof ᵏ þ grees clene, cowche fiſhe on chargeōs ꝫ cole the ſewe thorov a cloth onoward ꝫ ſūe it forth.

### Gele of Flefsh. .C. II.

Take ſwyn̄ feet ꝫ ſnowt̄ and the eerys ¹. capons. cōnyng̃ calū fete. ꝫ waſche hē clene. ꝫ do hē to ſeeþ in the þriddel ᵐ of wyne ꝫ vyneg̃ and wat̄ and make forth as bifore.

### Chyſanne ⁿ. .C. III.

Take Roches. hole Tench̄ and plays ꝫ ſmyte hem to gobett̄. fry hē ī oyle blānche almānd. fry hē ꝫ caſt p̄to raiſons corance make lyō of cruſt of brede of rede wyne ꝫ of vyneg̃ þ þridde part þw̄ ſyg̃ drawen ꝫ do p̄to powdō fort and ſalt. boile it. lay the Fiſhe ī an erthen panne caſt the ſewe p̄to. ſeeþ oynons ymynced ꝫ caſt þine. kepe hit and ete it colde.

ᵏ Dof, 1 e do of.
ˡ Lerys    Ears
ᵐ Thriddel. V. ad N° 67
ⁿ Chyſanne. Qu

Congur ᵒ in Sawſe.  .C. IIII.

Take the Cong̃ and ſcald hȳ. and ſmyte hȳ in pecys ⁊ ſeeþ hym. take pſel. mynt. peleṫ. roſmarye. ⁊ a litul ſawz̃e brede and ſalt, powdõ fort and a litel garlec, clow a lite, take and grynd it wel, drawe it up with vyneg̃ þurgh a cloth. caſt the fyſsh ĩ a veſſel and do þ ſewe onoward ⁊ s̃ue it forth.

Rygh ᵖ in Sawſe.  .C. V.

Take Ryghzes and make hem clene and do hẽ to ſeeþ. pyke hẽ clene and frye hem ĩ oile. take Almãnd and grynde hẽ ĩ waṫ or wyne, do þto almand blãnched hole fryed ĩ oile. ⁊ corãnce ſeeþ the lyõ grynde it ſmale ⁊ do þto garlec ygrõnde ⁊ litel ſalt ⁊ v̄ions powdõ fort ⁊ ſafron ⁊ boile it yfere, lay the Fyſshe in a veſſel and caſt the ſewe ĩto. and meſſe it forth colde.

Makerel in Sawſe.  .C. VI.

Take Makerels and ſmyte hem on pecys. caſt hem on waṫ and v̄ions ſeeþ hem with mynt and wiþ ooþ erbes, colõ it grene or zelow, and meſſe it forth.

---

ᵒ Congur. The Eel called *Congre Sawce*, Contents here, and Nᵒ 105, 106.

ᵖ Rygh. A Fiſh, and probably the *Ruffe*.

Pykes

### Pykes in brafey q. .C. VII.

Take Pykes and undo hem on þ womb ʳ and waifshe hem clene and lay hem on a rooft Irne ˢ þenne take gode wyne and powdͬ gyng ⁋ fug good wone ᵗ ⁋ falt, and boile it ĩ an erthen panne ⁋ meffe forth þ pyke ⁋ lay the fewe onoward.

### Porpeys in broth. .C. VIII.

Make as þou madeft Noumbles of Flefh with oynõns.

### Balloc ᵘ broth. .C. IX.

Take Eelys and hilde ˣ hem and kerue hem to pecys and do hem to feeþ in waī and wyne fo þat it be a litel oũ ftepid ʸ. do þto fawge and ooþ erbis w̄ few ᶻ oynõns ymynced, whan the Eelis buth foden ynowȝ do hem in a veffel, take a pyke and kerue it to gobett and feeþ hym in the fame broth do þto powdͬ gyng galyngale canel and pep, falt it and caft the Eelys þto ⁋ meffe it forth.

---

ᵠ Brafey. Qu.
ʳ Wombs. bellies.
ˢ rooft Irene. a roafting iron.
ᵗ good wone. a good deal V. Gloff
ᵘ Balloc. *Balloh*, Contents.
ˣ hilde. fkin.
ʸ on ftepid. fteeped therein. V Nº 110.
ᶻ few, i e. a few.

Eles

[ 54 ]

### Eles in Brewet. c. x.

Take Cruſt of brede and wyne and make a lyoꝛ, do þto oynoñs ymynced, powdoꝛ ¢ canel. ¢ a litel waꝉ and wyne. loke þat it be ſtepid, do þto ſalt, kerue þin Eelis ¢ feeþ hē wel and ſūe hem forth.

### Cawdel of Samōn. c. XI.

Take the guttꝗ of Samōn and make hem clene. pboile hem a lytell. take hem up and dyce hem. flyt the white of Lekes and kerue hem ſmale. cole the broth and do the lek þinne w̃ oile and lat it boile togyd yfere[a]. do the Samōn icorne þin, make a lyoꝛ of Almānd mylke ¢ of brede ¢ caſt þto ſpices, ſafron and ſalt, feeþ it wel. and loke þat it be not ſtondyng.

### Plays in Cyꝛee. c. XII.

Take Plays and ſmyte hem[b] to pecys and fry hem in oyle. drawe a lyoꝛ of brede ¢ gode broth ¢ vynegꝝ. and do jto powdoꝛ gyng. canel. pep and ſalt and loke þ it be not ſtondyng.

### For to make Flaumpeyns. c. XIII.

Take clene pork and boile it tendre. þenne hewe it ſmall and bray it ſmal in a morꝉ. take fyg and boile

---

[a] togyd yfere One of theſe ſhould be ſtruck out.
[b] Vide Nº 10.. Qu.

hem

hem tendre ln smale ale. and bray hem and tendre chese ꝑwith. þēne waisthe hem ĩ wat͛ ꝯ þene lyͬ ͨ hem alle togiͩdͭ w Ayreñ, þenne taᴋe powdͬo of pep. or els powdͬo marchãnt ꝯ ayreñ and a porcion of safroñ and salt. þeñe take blank sugͬ. eyreñ ꝯ floͬ ꝯ make a past w ͭa roller, þene make ꝑof smale pelettͩ. ꝯ fry hē broũ ĩ clene grece ꝯ set hem asyde. þenne make of þͭ oopͬ deel ͤ of þ past long coffyns ͬ ꝯ do þ comade ͬ þͬin. and close hē fane with a coutͬo ͪ, ꝯ pynche hē smale about. þãne kyt aboue foure oꝑ sex wayes, þanne take eũyͥ of þͭ kuttyng up, ꝯ þeñe colͭo it w zolkes of Ayreñ, and plãnt hem thick, ĩto the flaumpeyns above þͬ þͬ kutteʃt hē ꝯ set hēĩ an ovene and lat hem bake esclichͨ. and þanne sũe hem forth.

For to make Noumblͬ in Lent. .c. xiiii.

Take the blode of pykes oꝑ of congͬ and nymeͥ the paũnch of pykes. of congͬ and of grete code lyngᵐ, ꝯ

---

ͨ ifͬ mix.
ͩ Pelettes Pel'ʒͭ, Ms Ed Nᵒ 16 Balls, pellets, from Fr. *pelote*.
ͤ decl deal, 1 c part, hạlt
ͬ Coffyns. Pies without lids.
ᴢ comade Qu.
ͪ coutͬo coverture, a lid. ͥ eũj. every.
ᴋ eselich. easily, gently.
ͥ nyme. take. Perpetually used in Ms. Ed. from Sax. niman.
ᵐ code lyng If a Codling be a *small cod*, as we now understand it, *great codling* seems a contradiction in terms.

4 boile

boile hē tendre ⁊ mynce hē ſmale ⁊ do hē ĩ þat blode. take cruſt of white brede ⁊ ſtỹne it thurgh a cloth. þenne take oynoñs iboiled and mynced. take pep and ſafroñ. wyne. vyneg ayſell ⁿ oþ aleg̃ ⁊ do þto ⁊ sũe forth.

For to make Chawdon ᵒ for Lent.   .c. xv.

Take blode of gurnard and cong̃ ⁊ þ panch of gurnard and boile hē tendre ⁊ mynce hē ſmale, and make a lyre of white Cruſt and oynons ymynced, bray it ĩ a mort ⁊ þanne boile it togyd til it be ſtondyng. þenne take vyneg oþ ayſell ⁊ ſafroñ ⁊ put it þto and sũe it forth.

Furmente with Porpeys.   .c. xvi.

Take clene whete and bete it ſmall in a mort and fanne out clene the douſt, þenne waiſthe it clene and boile it tyl it be tendre and broũ. þanne take the ſecunde mylk of Almãnd ⁊ do þto. boile hē togyd til it be ſtondyng, and take þ firſt mylke ⁊ alye it up wiþ a peñe ᵖ. take up the porpays out of the Furmente ⁊ leſne hem ĩ a diſhe with hoot waṱ. ⁊ do ſafroñ

---

ⁿ Ayſell. L.'ei, vinegar Litdeton.
ᵒ Chawdon V. Gloſſ.
ᵖ Penre Feather, or p.n. Mſ. Ed. 28.

to þe furmente. and if the porpays be salt. seeþ it by hy͂ self, and sue͂ it forth.

Fylett9 in galyntyne. .c.xvii.

Take Pork, and rost it tyl the blode be tryed out ⁊ þe broth[q]. take crust9 of brede and bray hem ĩ a mort͂, ā drawe hē thurgh a cloth with þe broth, þenne take oy-nons ā leshe hem on brede ā do to the broth. þanne take pork, and leshe it clene with a dressyng knyf and cast it into þe pot broth, ⁊ lat it boile til it be more tendre. þanne take þat lyō þ9to. þāne take a porciō of pep and sandr9 ⁊ do þ9to. þanne take psel ⁊ ysope ⁊ mynce it smāle ⁊ do þ9to. þāne take rede wyne oþ9 white grece ⁊ raysons ⁊ do þ9to. ⁊ lat it boile a lytel.

Veel in buknade[r]. .c.xviii.

Take fayr Veel and kyt it in smale pecys and boile it tendre ĩ fyne broth oþ9 in wat͂. þanne take white brede oþ9 wastel[s], and drawe þ9of a white . . . . lyō wiþ fyne broth, and do þe lyō to the Veel, ⁊ do safron þ9to, þāne take p͛sel ⁊ bray it ĩ a mort͂ ⁊ the Juys[t] þ9of do þ9to, and þāne is þis half zelow ⁊ half grene.

[q] the broth. Suppo'ed to be prepared beforehand.
[r] Buknade. V N° 17.
[s] Wastel. V Gloss.
[t] Juys. Juice

þāne take a porcion̄ of wyne ⁊ powdᵒ marchant ⁊ do þto and lat it boile wele, and do þto a litel of ᵘ vyneg̃. ⁊ sūe forth.

## Sooles in Cynee ˣ.   .C. XIX.

Take Sooles and hylde hem, feeþ hem in waī, fmyte hē on pecys and take away the fynnes take oyroñs ıboıled ⁊ grynde the fynn p̄w and brede, draᵣe it up with the felf broth. do þto powdᵒ fort, fafroñ ⁊ hony clarified with falt, feeþ it alle yfere. broıle the fooles ⁊ meffe it ī dyfsh ⁊ lay the fewe above. ⁊ sūe forth.

## Tench in Cyñec.   XXVI.

Take Tench and fmyte hem to pecys, fry hem, drawe a lyo of Rayfons corañce witþ wyne and waī, do þto Lool raıfons ⁊ powdᵒ of gyng̃ of clowes of canel of pep do the Tench þto ⁊ feeþ hē w fug̃ cypre ⁊ falt. ⁊ meffe forth.

---

ᵘ litel of vyneg' We fay, *a little vinegar*, omitting *of*. So 152, *a ball of lard*.

ˣ Cynee *C. ij.*, Contents, both here and Nº 120. 123. See before, Nº 25.

Oyſters in Gravey. XX. V. I.

Schyl ʸ Oyſters and ſeeþ hem in wyne and in haie ᶻ own broth cole the broth thurgh a cloth. take almand blanched, grynde hē and drawe hē up with the ſelf broth. ⁊ alye it wiþ flo of Rys. and do the oyſters þinne, caſt in powdʳ of gyng, ſug, macys. ſeeþ it not to ſtondyng and ſue forth.

Muſkels ᵃ in brewet. XX. VI. II.

Take muſkels, pyke hem, ſeeþ hem with the owne broth, make a lyo of cruſt ᵇ ⁊ vyneg do in oynons mynced. ⁊ caſt the muſkels þto ⁊ ſeeþ it. ⁊ do þto powdʳ w ͭ a lytel ſalt ⁊ ſafron the ſamewiſe make of oyſters.

Oyſters in Cynee. XX. VI III.

Take Oyſters pboile hem ĩ her owne broth, make a lyo of cruſt of brede ⁊ drawe it up wiþ the broth and vyneg mynce oynons ⁊ do þto with erbes. ⁊ caſt the oyſters þinne. boile it. ⁊ do þto powdʳ fort ⁊ ſalt. ⁊ meſſe it forth.

ʸ Schyl    ſhell, take of the ſhells
ᶻ haie. their   *her*   N° 123   Chaucer.
ᵃ Muſkles   *muſkels* below, and the Contents.   Muſcles.
ᵇ cruſtes, i. e. of bread.

Cawdel

### Cawdel of Muſkels. XX. VI. IIII.

Take and ſeeþ muſkels, pyke hem clene, and waiſshe hem clene ĩ wyne. take almand ҉ bray hẽ. take sõme of the muſkels and grynde hẽ. ҉ ſome hewe ſmale, drawe the muſkels ygrõnd w̃ the ſelf broth. wryng the almãnd with faire waẽ. do alle þiſe togid. do þto vious and vyneg. take whyte of lek ҉ pboile hẽ wel. wryng oute the waẽ and hewe hẽ ſmale. caſt oile þto w̃ oynonẽ pboiled ҉ mynced ſmale do þto powdõ fort, ſafroñ and ſalt. a lytel ſeeþ it not to to ᵉ ſtondyng ҉ meſſe it forth.

### Mortrews of Fyſsh. XX VI. V.

Take codlyng, haddok, oþ hake and lynõs with the rawnes ᵈ and ſeeþ it wel in waẽ. pyke out þͤ bones, gryndē ſmale the Fyſshe, drawe a lyõ of almãnd ҉ brede w̃ the ſelf broth. and do the Fyſshe gronden þto. and ſeeþ it and do þto powdõ fort, ſafroñ and ſalt, and make it ſtondyng.

### Laumpreys in galyntyne. XX VI. VI.

Take Laumpreys and ſle ᵉ hem with vyneg oþ with white wyne ҉ ſalt, ſcalde hẽ ĩ waẽ. ſlyt hem a litel

---

ᶜ o to, . e too too    Vide Nᵒ 17.
ᵈ rawnes. roes.         ᵉ ſle. flay, kll.

[ 61 ]

at þ nauel. . . . . . . ⁊ reſt a litel at the nauel. take out the gutt at the ende. kepe wele the blode. put the Laumprey on a ſpyt. rooſt hỹ ⁊ kepe wel the grece. grynde rayſons of corance. hỹ up ᶠw vyneḡ. wyne. and cruſt of brede. do þto powdo͛ of gynḡ. of galyngale ᵍ. flo͛ of canel. powdo͛ of clow. and do þto raiſons of corance hoole. w þ blode ⁊ þ grece. ſeeþ it ⁊ ſalt it, boile it not to ſtondyng, take up the Laumprey do hỹ in a chargeo͛ ʰ, ⁊ lay þ ſewe onoward, ⁊ ſuͤ hỹ forth.

### Laumpions in galyntyne.    XX VI. VII.

Take Lamprons and ſcalde hē. ſeeþ hem, meng powdo͛ galyngale and ſome of the broth togyd ⁊ boile it ⁊ do þto powdo͛ of gyng ⁊ ſalt. take the Laumprons ⁊ boile hē ⁊ lay hē i dyſh. ⁊ lay the ſewe above. ⁊ ſuͤ fort.

### Loſeyns ⁱ in Fyſsh Day.    XX VI. VIII.

Take Almand unblanched and waſſthe hē clene, drawe hē up with wat. ſeeþ þ mylke ⁊ alȝe it up w

---

ᶠ hỹ up  A word ſeems omitted, *drawe* or *lye*.
ᵍ of galyngale, i e powder. V Nᵒ 101.
ʰ Chargeo'. charger or diſh. V Nᵒ 127.
ⁱ Loſeyns, *Lofyns*, Contents.

loſeyns.

loſeyns. caſt p̛to ſafroñ. ſug̃. ⁊ ſalt ⁊ meſſe it forth with colyandre ĩ confyt rede, ⁊ sũe it forth.

### Sowp̛ of galyntyne [k].     xx VI. IX.

Take powdo͛ of galyngale with ſug̃ and ſalt and boile it yfere. take brede ytoſted. and lay the ſewe onoward. and sũe it forth.

### Sobre Sawſe.     xx VI. X.

Take Rayſoñs, grynde hem with cruſtꝯ of brede, and drawe it up with wyne. do p̛to gode powdo͛s and ſalt. and ſeep̛ it. fry rochꝯ, loochꝯ, foolꝯ, op̛ oop̛ gode Fyſh, caſt p̛ ſewe above, ⁊ sũe it forth.

### Cold Brewet.     xx VI XI.

Take crome [l] of almañdꝯ. dry it in a cloth. and whan it is dryed do it in a veſſel, do p̛to ſalt, ſug̃, and white powdo͛ of gyng̃ and Juys of Fenel and wyne. and lat it wel ſtonde. lay full ⁊ meſſe ⁊ dreſſe it forth.

### Peerꝯ [m] in confyt.     xx VI XII.

Take peerꝯ and pare hẽ clene. take gode rede wyne ⁊ mulberes [n] op̛ ſañdrꝯ and ſeep̛ p̛ peerꝯ p̛in ⁊ whan þei

---

[k] Sowpes of Galyntyre. Contents has *in*, recte. *Sowpes* means Sops.    [l] crome crumb, pulp.    [m] Peerꝯ pears.    [n] mulberes. mulberr es, for colouring.

buth

buþ yſode, take hē up, make a ſyryp of wyne greke, oþ vnage º w blañche powdᵈ oþ white ſug̃ and powdõ gyng̃ ⁊ do the per̃ þin. ſeeþ it a lytel ⁊ meſſe it forth.

### Egurdouce ᴾ of Fyſhe.    xx. VI. XIII.

Take Loch oþ Tench oþ Solys ſmyte hem on pecys, fry hē in oyle. take half wyne half vyneg̃ and ſug̃ ⁊ make a ſiryp. do þto oynoñs icorue ᑫ raiſoñs corañce. and grete rayſoñs. do þto hole ſpices. gode powdõs and ſalt. meſſe þ fyſh ⁊ lay þ ſewe aboue and sūe forth.

### Colde Brewet.    xx VI. XIIII.

Take Almañd and grynde hē. take the tweydel ʳ of wyne oþ the þriddell of vyneg̃. drawe up the Almañd þw̃. take anys ſug̃ ⁊ branch of fenel grene a fewe. ⁊ drawe hē up togȳd w þ mylke take poudõ of canell. of gyng̃. clow. ⁊ maces hoole. take kydde oþ chikeñs oþ fleſsh. ⁊ choppe hem ſmall and ſeeþ hem. take all þis fleſh whan it is ſodeñ ⁊ lay it ī a

---

º Vernage. Vernaccia, a ſort of Italian white wine. V. Gloſſ
ᴾ Egurdouce. Vide Gloſſ.
ᑫ icorue, icorven. cut. V. Gloſſ.
ʳ Tweydel. Two parts.

clene

clene veſſel & boile þ͡ f̾re & caſt ͥto ſalt. þenne caſt al þis in þ͡ pot with fleſh. &c.ˢ

Pevorat ͭ for Veel and Venyſon. VI. XV.

Take Brede & fry it in grece. drawe it up with broth and vyneg̾, take ͥto powd͡͡ of pep & ſalt and ſette it on the fyre. boile it and meſſe it forth.

Sawſe ᵘ blanche for Capons yſode. VI. XVI.

Take Almand blanched and grynd hem al to douſt. temp it up with vions and powd͡͡ of gyngyn and meſſe it forth.

Sawſe Noyre for Capons yroſted. VI. XVII.

Take the lyu of Capons and rooſt it wel. take anyſe and greynes de Parys ˣ. gyng. canel. & a lytill cruſt of brede and gnde it ſmale. and grynde it up w vions. and with grece of Capons. boyle it and ſue it forth.

ˢ &c. i. e. ſue forth

ᵗ Pevorat. Pererade, from the pepper of which it is principally compoſed.

ᵘ Sawſe. Sauce, Contents. As Nº 137.

ˣ de Parys. Cf. Paradiſe. V. Pref.

Galyntyne.

### Galyntyne[y]. VI. XVIII.

Take crust of Brede and grynde hem smale, do þto powdõ of galyngale, of canel, of gyngyn and salt it, tempre it with vyneg and drawe it up þurgh a straynõ & messe it forth.

### Gyngeñ[z]. VI. XIX.

Take payndemayn and pare it clene and funde it in Vineg, grynde it and temp it wiþ Vyneg, and with powdõ gyng and salt, drawe it thurgh a styno. and sue forth.

### Verde[a] Sawse. XX. VII.

Take psel. mynt. garlek. a litul spell[b] and sawge, a litul canel. gyng. pip. wyne. brede. vyneg & salt grynde it imal w̃ safroñ & messe it forth.

### Sawse Noyre for Malard. XX. VII. I.

Take brede and blode iboiled. and grynde it and drawe it thurgh a cloth w̃ Vyneg, do þto powdõ of

---

[y] Galyntyne   Galentyne, Contents

[z] Gyngeñ   From the powder of Ginger therein used.

[a] Verde.   It has the sound of *Green-sauce*, but as there is no Sorel in it, it is so named from the other herbs.

[b] 1 litul Spell.   Wild thyme

gyng ad of pep. ⁊ þ grece of the Maulard. falt it. boile it wel and sue it forth.

### Cawdel for Gees. XX VII. II.

Take garlec and gnde it fmale. Safron and flo þ- with ⁊ falt. and temp it up with Cowe Mylke. and feeþ it wel and sue it forth.

### Chawdon ᶜ for Swann. XX VII. III.

Take þ lyu and þ offall ᵈ of the Swann ⁊ do it to feeþ ī gode broth. take it up. take out þ bonys. take ⁊ hewe the flefsh fmale. make a Lyo of crust of brede ⁊ of þ blode of þ Swan yfoden. ⁊ do þto powdo of clow ⁊ of pip ⁊ of wyne ⁊ falt, ⁊ feeþ it ⁊ caft þ flefsh þto ihewed. and meffe it forth w̄ þ Swan.

### Sawfe Camelyne ᵉ. XX. VII. IIII.

Take Rayfons of Corance. ⁊ kyrnels of notys. ⁊ crust of brede ⁊ powdo of gyng clow flo of canel. by it ᶠ wel togyd and do it þto. falt it, temp it up with vyneg. and sue it forth.

---

ᶜ Chawdōn. V. Gloff.
ᵈ offall. *Exta*, Gibles.
ᵉ Camelyne. Qu. if *Camelyne* from the *Fluor of Canel*?
ᶠ by bray.

Lumbard

[ 67 ]

Lumbard Muſtard.     XV VII. V.

Take Muſtard ſeed and waſhe it & drye it ĩ an ovene, grynde it drye. ſaiſe it thurgh a ſarſe. clarifie hony w̃ wyne & vyneg & ſtere it wel togedr and make it thikke ynow. & whan þu wilt ſpende þof make it thynne w̃ wyne.

Nota.     XX. VII. VI.

Cranes [g] and Heroñs ſhul be armed [h] with lard of Swyne. and eten with gyng.

Nota.     XX VII. VII.

Pokok and Ptruch ſhul be pboiled. lardid and roſted. and eten with gyngen.

---

[g] Cranes. A diſh frequent formerly at great tables. Archæologia, II. p. 171. mentioned with Herons, as here, Mſ. Ed. 3. where the ſame Recipe occurs. et v. Lel. Coll. IV. p. 226 VI. p. 38. Rabelais, IV. c 59 E. of Devon's Feaſt.

[h] armed. Mſ. Ed. Nº 3 has enarmed, as may be read there. Exarmed, however, in Lel Collect. IV p. 225 means, decorated with coate of arms Sheldes of Brawn are there *in armor*, p. 226. However, there is ſuch a word as enorned. Leland, p. 280 285. 297. which approaches nearer.

[ 68 ]

### Fry blanched.     VII. VIII.

Take Almand blanched and grynde hē al to douſt, do þiſe ī a thynne foile. cloſe it þinne faſt. and fry it in Oile. clarifie hony w̄ Wyne. & bake it þw̄

### Frytō of Paſternak of of Apples¹.     VII. IX.

Take ſkyrwat and paſtnak and apples, & pboile hē, make a batō of flō and ayreñ, caſt þto ale. ſafroñ & ſalt. wete hē ī þ batō and frye hē ī oile or ī grece. do þto Almañd Mylk. & ſue it forth.

### Frytō of Mylke.     VII. X.

Take of crudd ᵏ and p̄ſſe out þ wheyze¹. do þto ſū whyte of ayreñ. fry hē. do þto. & lay on ſug and meſſe forth.

### Frytō of Erbes.     VII. XI.

Take gode erbys. grynde hē and medle ᵐ hē w̄ flō and wat̄ & a lytel zeſt and ſalt, and frye hē ī oyle. and ete hē w clere hony.

---

¹ Frytour, &c. Contents has only *Fry'ours of Paſternakes*. N. B. *Fry'our* is *Fritter*.

ᵏ Cruddes. Curds per metatheſia.

ˡ wheyze whey.      ᵐ medle. m v.

Raſyols.

[ 69 ]

### Rasyols ⁿ.   XX. VII. XII.

Take swyne lyuos and seeþ hē wel. take brede & grate it. and take zolkes of ayren & make hit sowple ᵒ and do þto a lytull of lard carnōn lyche a dee ᵖ. chese gtyd ᵍ & whyte grece. powdo douce & of gyng & wynde it to ball ʳ as grete as apples. take þ calle of þᵉ swyne & cast eue ˢ by hȳ self þin. Make a Crust ī a trape ᵗ. and lay þ ball þin & bake it. and whan þey buth ynowʒ: put þin a layo of ayren w powdo fort and Safron. and sue it forth.

### Whyte Mylat ᵘ.   XX. VII. XIII.

Take Ayren and wryng hē thurgh a cloth. take powdo fort, brede igrated, & safron, & cast þto a gode qntite of vyneg with a litull salt, medle all yfere. make a foile ī a trap & bake it wel þinne. and sue it forth.

ⁿ Rasyols. Rasiowls, Contents. Qu the etymcn.

ᵒ sowple. supple

ᵖ carnōn lyche a dee. Cut like dice, diced. Fr. *Dé*, singular of *Dice*

ᵍ gtyd. grated. *igrated*, Nº 153.

ʳ wynde it to balles. make it into Balls.

ˢ eue. each.

ᵗ trape. pan, or dish. French

ᵘ Mylates. Contents, *Miletes*, but 155 as here. Qu.

### Cruſtard ˣ of Fleſh.   XXVII. XIIII.

Take peions ʸ and ſmale bridd ſmyte hē ĩ gobett wiþ ꝯiaws ᶻ do þto ſaffroñ, make a cruſt ĩ a trap. and pynche it. ⁊ cowche þ fleſh þinne. ⁊ caſt þinne Raiſons corance. powdō douce and ſalt. breke ayreñ and wryng hem thurgh a cloth ⁊ ſwyng þ ſewe of þ ꝯi.w and helde it ᵃ upon the fleſh. coūe it ⁊ bake it wel. and ſūe it forth.

### Mylat of Pork.   XXVII. XV.

Hewe Pork al to pecys and medle it w ayreñ ⁊ cheſe igted. do þto powdō fort ſafroñ ⁊ pyner ᵇ with ſalt, make a cruſt ĩ a trap, bake it wel þinne, and ſūe it forth.

### Cruſtard of Fyſshe.   XXVII. XVI.

Take loch, laumproñs, and Eelis. ſmyte hem on pecys, and ſtewe hē wiþ Almañd Mylke and ꝯions, frye the loch ĩ oile as tofore. and lay þ fiſh þinne.

---

ˣ Cruſtards. Pies.
ʸ peions. pigeons. V. ad Nº 48.
ᶻ ꝯiaws. Verjuice
ᵃ helde it. pour, caſt.
ᵇ pyner. Vide Pref.

caſt

[ 71 ]

caſt þon powdō fort powdō douce. with rayſons corañce & prunes damyſyns. take galyntyn and þ ſewe þinne, and ſwyng it togȳd and caſt ĩ the trape. & bake it and ſūe it forth.

Cruſtard of Eerbis ᵉ on fyſsh Day.　xx. vii. xvii.

Take gode Eerbys and grynde hē ſmale with wallenot pyked clene. a grete portioñ. lye it up almoſt wiþ as myche ⁱons as waͭt. ſeeþ it wel w̄ powdō and Safroñ woͭute Salt. make a cruſt in a tra͞p and do þ fyſsh þinne unſtewed wiþ a litel oile & gode Powdō. whan it is half ybake do þ ſewe þto & bake it up. If þᵘ wilt make ‧t clere of Fyſsh ſeeþ ayreñ harde. & take out þ zolk & gⁱnde hē w̄ gode powdōs. and alye it up with gode ſtewes ᵈ and ſūe it forth.

Leſshes ᵉ fryed in lenton ᶠ.　xx. vii. xviii.

Drawe a thick almande Mylke wiþ waͭt. take daͭ and pyke hē clene w̄ apples and peer & mynce hē w̄ ᵖnes damyſyns. take out þ ſtoⁿ out of þ ᵖnes. & kerue the ᵖnes a two. do þto Raiſons ſug. flō of canel. hoole macys and clow. gode powdōs & ſalt. colō

---

ᵉ Erbis. Rather *Erbis and Fyſh*
ᵈ ſtewes V Nᵒ 170
ᵉ Leſhes V Leche Lumbard in Gloſſ.
ᶠ lenton. Lentōn, Contents, i e Lent

hem

hem up w͛ sandr̊. meng þise w th oile, make a coffyn as þ͞ didest bifor̄ ⁊ do þis Fars ᵍ þin. and bake it wel and sūe it forth.

### Wastels yfarced.     VII. XIX.ˣˣ

Take a Wastel and hewe out þ crūnnes. take ayren ⁊ shepis talow ⁊ þ crinn of þ same Wastell powd͛ fort ⁊ salt w Safron and Raisons corance. ⁊ medle alle þise ɣfere ⁊ do it in þ Wastel. close it ⁊ bynde it fast togidre. and seeþ it wel.

### Sawge yfarced.     VIII.ˣˣ

Take sawge. grynde it and temp it up with ayren. ⁊ sawcyst ʰ ⁊ kerf hȳ to gobett and cast it ī a possynet. and do þwiþ grece ⁊ frye it. Whan it is fryed ynowz cast þto sawge w ayren make it not to harde. cast þto powd͛ douce, messe it forth. If it be in Ymber day take sauge butt ⁊ ayren. and lat it stonde wel by þ sause ⁱ, ⁊ sūe it forth.

### Sawgeat ᵏ.     VIII. L.ˣˣ

Take Pork and seeþ it wel and gnde it smale and medle it wiþ ayren ⁊ brede. ygrated. do þto powd͛

---

ᵍ F r.. V le G'off.      ʰ sawcyster. Qu.
ⁱ Stonde wel by the sause. Become thick with the sauce.
ᵏ Sawgeat. So named from the Sage, or Sawge.

fort

[ 73 ]

fort and safroñ with pyñ & salt. take & close litull Ba'l ĩ foiles¹ of sawge. wete it with a batõ of ayıen & fry it. & sũe it forth.

### Cryspes ᵐ.     XX. VIII. II.

Take flõ of pandemayn and medle it with white grece oũ the fyr in a chawfõⁿ and do the batõ þto queıntlich ᵒ þurgh þy fyngõs. or thurgh a skymõ. and lat it a litul ᵖ quayle ᵠ a litell so þ þ be hool þinne. And if þ wilt colõ it wiþ alkenet ysoñdyt. take hẽ up & cast þinne sug, and sũe hẽ forth.

### Cryspels.     XX VIII. III.

Take and make a foile of gode Past as thynne as Pap. keruc it out & fry it in oile. oþ, ĩ þʳ grece and

---

¹ foiles   leaves.

ᵐ Cryspes. Ms. Ed. Nº 26. *Cryppys*, meaning *Crups*, Chaucer having *crips*, by transposition, for *crisp*. In Kent *p* is commonly put before the *s*, as *haps* is *hasp*, *waps* is *wasp*. V. Junius. V. *Happs*, and *Haspe*, and *Wasp*.

ⁿ chawfõ. chaffing dish.
ᵒ quentlich'. nicely.
ᵖ a litul. Dele.
ᵠ quayle. an cool?
ʳ þ grece. Dele *the*.

K                       þ re-þ remnant ˢ, take hony clarified and flaunne ᵗ þw, alye hem up and sue hem forth.

## Tartee.     XX VIII. IIII.

Take pork ysode. hewe it & bray it. do þto ayren. Raisons sug and powdo of gyng. powdo douce. and smale bridd þamong & white grece. take prunes, safron. & salt, and make a crust i a trap & do þ Fars ᵘ þin. & bake it wel & sue it forth.

## Tart in Ymbre ˣ day.     XX VIII. V.

Take and pboile Oynons psse out þ wat & hewe he smale. take brede & bray it i a mort. and temp it up w Ayren. do þto butt safron and salt. & raisons corans. & a litel sug with powdo douce. and bake it i a trap. & sue it forth.

## Tart de Bry ʸ.     X VIII. VI.

Take a Crust ynche depe in a trap. take zolkes of Ayren rawe & chese ruayn ᶻ. & medle it & þ zolkes to-

---

ˢ þ remnant, i e as for the remnant  
ᵗ flaunne. French *flan*, custard.  
ᵘ þ Fars, r. þ Fars.  
ˣ Ymbre   Ember  
ʸ de Bry   Qu. *Bre*, the country.  
ᶻ Chese ruayn. Qu. of Rouen. V. ad 49.

gyd.

gyd. and do þto powdo gyng. sug. safron. and salt. do it in a trap, bake it and sue it forth.

### Tart de brymlent [a].  xx.VIII.VII.

Take Fyg & Raysons. & waisshe hē in Wyne. and gnde hem smale wt apples & per clene ypiked. take hē up and cast hē in a pot wiþ wyne and sug. take salwar Salmōn [b] ysode. oþ codlyng, oþ haddok, & bray hē smal. & do þto white powdos & hool spices. & salt. and seeþ it. and whanne it is sode ynowȝ. take it up and do it in a vessel and lat it kele. make a Coffyn an ynche depe & do þ fars þin. Plant it boue [c] wt prunes and damysyns. take þ ston out, and wiþ dates q̄rte rede [d] and piked clene. and coūe the coffyn, and bake it wel, and sue it forth.

### Tartes of Flesh [e].  xx.VIII.VIII.

Take Pork ysode and grynde it smale. tarde [f] harde

---

[a] Brymlent. Perhaps Midlent or High Lent. *Bryme*, in Cotgrave, is the *midst* of Winter. The fare is certainly lenten. A.S. bryme Solennis, or beginning of Lent, from A.S. brymm, ora, margo. Yet, after all, it may be a mistake for *Prymlent*.

[b] salwar Samōn. V. ad Nº 98.

[c] plant it above. Stick it *above*, or on the top.

[d] q̄rte red quartered

[e] Tartes of Flesh. So we have *Tarte Poleyn*, Lel. Coll. IV. p 226. i.e. of Pullen, or Poultry.

[f] tarde, r. *take*. For see Nº 169.

eyren ısode ҭ ygronde and do þto with Chefe ygronde. take gode powdo and hool spices, sug, safron, and salt ҭ do þto. make a coffyn as to feel sayde ᵍ ҭ do þis jnne, ҭ plant it wᵗ smale bridd istyned ҭ conyng. ҭ hewe hē to smale gobett ҭ bake it as tofore. ҭ sue it forth.

### Tartlet.     XX VIII. IX.

Take Veel ysode and gnde it smale. take harde Eyren ısode and ygrond ҭ do þto with prunes hoole ʰ. dat. ıcorue pyn and Raısons corance. hool spices ҭ powdo. sug salt, and make a litell coffyn and do þis fars jnne. ҭ bake it ҭ sue it forth.

### Tart of Fysshe.     XX VIII. X.

Take Eelys and Samon and smyte hē on pecys. ҭ stewe it ĩ almand mylke and vious. drawe up on almand mylk wiþ þ stewe. Pyke out the bon clene of þ fyısh. aᵈ save þ myddell pece hoole of þ Eelys ҭ gnde þ coþ fiısh smale. and do þto powdo, sug, ҭ salt and gted brede. ҭ fors þ Eelys j w þer as ᵏ þ borys were medle þ ooþ dele of the fars ҭ þ mylk togıd. and colo

---

ᵍ o feel sayde. perhaps, *to hola t'e fame.*
ʰ hoole, v ho'e
ⁱ . rather *les*, i. e. them
ᵏ fers. where. V. Nº 177.

it

[ 77 ]

it wt ſañdr̉. make a cruſt in a trap̄ as before. and bake it þın and sūe ıt forth.

### Sambocade [1].  xx VIII. XI.

Take and make a Cruſt ī a trap̄. ꝫ take a crudd̉ and wryng out þ wheyze. and dıawe hē þurgh̄ a ſtÿnd̉. and put ī þ ſtÿnd̉ cruſt. do p̄to ſug̃ the þrıdde part ꝫ ſomdel [m] whyte of Ayreñ. ꝫ ſhake þın blom̃ of elren [n]. ꝫ bake it up wt curoſe [o] ꝫ meſſe ıt forth.

### Erbolat̉ [p].  xx VIII. XII.

Take p̄ſel, mynt̉ [q], ſauey, ꝫ ſauge, tanſey, vuayn̉, clarry, rewe, dıtayn, fenel, ſouthrenwode, hewe hē ꝫ gnde hē ſmale, medle hē up wt Ayreñ. do butt ī a tıap̄. ꝫ do þ fars p̄to. ꝫ bake it ꝫ meſſe ıt forth.

### Nyſebek [r].  xx VIII. XIII.

Take þe þrıdde paıt of ſowre Dokk̉ and flō p̄to. ꝫ bete it toged tyl ıt be as towh as eny lyme. caſt p̄to

---

[1] Sambucade   As made of the *Sambucus*, or Elder.

[m] Somdel   Some

[n] Blom of Elren   Elder flowers.

[o] curoſe

[p] Erbolat, ı. e. Herbolade, a confection of herbs.

[q] myntes, mint.

[r] Nyſebek   Qu.

ſalt.

[ 78 ]

falt. ⁊ do it ĩ a difshe holke ˢ in þ̆ bothom, and let it out wiþ þy fingͭ queynchche ᵗ ĩ a chowfer ᵘ wiþ oile. ⁊ frye it wel. and whan it is ynowȝ. take it out and caſt p̄to fugͭ ⁊c.

For to make Pom̄e Dorryle ˣ and oþ̄ e þyng. VIII.XIIII.

Take þ̆ lire of Pork rawe. and giynde it fmale. medle it up wiþ powdre fort, fafroñ, and falt, and do p̄to Raifoп̄s of Corañce, make baȗ þ̄of. and wete it wele ĩ white of ayreñ ⁊ do it to feeþ ĩ boıllȳg waƚ. take hem up and put hem on a fpyt. roſt hē wel and take pſel ygronde and wryng it up with ayren ⁊ a pty of flo. and lat erne ʸ abonte þ̆ fpyt. And if þ̆ wılt, take for pſel fafroñ, and sūe it forth.

ˢ holke  Qu. hollow
ᵗ queynchche  an *queyntlıcb'*, as N° 162.
ᵘ Chowfer.  chaffing difh, as N° 162

ˣ Pom̄e dorryle.  Contents, *p̄ɔ dorryes*, rectè, for MS Ed 4:, has *Pommedorry*; and fee N° 171. So named from the *balls* and *the gıldıng*. " Pommes dorées, golden apples " Cotgrave. *Pōndorrey*. MS. Ed. 58; but vide *Dorry* in Gloff.

ʸ erne.  Qu.

Cotagres

### Cotagres [z]. XXVIII. XV.

Take and make þ self fars [a]. but do ꝯto pyn and sug̃. take an hole rowsted cok, pulle hȳ [b] ⁊ hylde [c] hym al togyd̃ saue þ legg̃. take a pigg and hilde [d] hȳ fro þ mydd doūward, fylle hī ful of þ fars ⁊ sowe hȳ fast togid. do hȳ in a panne ⁊ seeþ hȳ wel. and whan þei bene isode, do hē on a spyt ⁊ rost it wele. colo͞ꝛ it w̃ zolkes of ayren and safron̄, lay ꝯon foyles [e] of gold and of silū. and sūe hit forth.

### Hert rowee [f]. XXVIII. XVI.

Take þ mawe of þ grete Swyne. and fyse oꝯ sex of pigg̃ mawe. fyll hē full of þ self fars. ⁊ sowe hē fast, ꝑboile hē. take hē up ⁊ make smale prews [g] of gode past and frye hē. take þese prews yfryed ⁊ seeþ [h]

---

[z] Cotagres. This is a sumptuous dish. Perhaps we should read *Cokagres*, from the *cock* and *grees*, or wild pig, therein used. V. *vyne grace* in Gloss.

[a] self fars. Same as preceding Recipe.

[b] pulle hȳ, i. e. in pieces.

[c] hylde cast

[d] hilde. skin

[e] foyles. leaves, of Laurel or Bay, suppose, gilt and silvered for ornament.

[f] Hert rowee. Contents, *Hart rows*; perhaps from *heart*.

[g] prews. Qu V. in Gloss.

[h] seeþ. There is a fault here, it means *stick*.

hē

[ 80 ]

hē þicke iu þ̃ mawͨ on þ̃ fars made aftͭ¹ an urchoñ woute leggͭ put hem on a fpyt ⁊ rooſt hē ⁊ coloͬ hem wͭ fafroñ ⁊ meſſe hē forth.

Potews ᵏ.    XX VIII. XVII.

Take Pottͦ of Erþ lytellͨ of half a quart and fyll hem full of fars of poͬme dorryes ¹. oþ̃ make wɪth þyn honde. oþ̃ ĭ a moolde pottͦ of þ̃ felf fars put hem ĭ watͭ ⁊ feeþ hē up wel. and whan þey buth ynowȝ. breke þ̃ pott of erþ ⁊ do þ̃ fars on þ̃ fpyt ⁊ roſt hē wel. and whan þeɪ buth yrofted. coloͬ hem as pōme dorryes. make of lɪtull prewes ᵐ gode paſt, fɪye hem oþ̃ roſt hem wel ĭ grece. ⁊ make þ̃ of Eerys ⁿ to pottͦ ⁊ coloͬ it. and make rofys ᵒ of gode paſt, ⁊ frye hē, ⁊ put þ̃ ſteles ᵖ ĭ þ̃ hole þ̃ ᑫ þ̃ fpyt was. ⁊ coloͬ ɪt with whyte. oþ̃ rede. ⁊ ſue it forth.

ᵃ after,  ᵉ lɪke
ᵏ Potews   probably from the *pots* employed.
¹ pōme dorryes. Vide ad Nº 174.
ᵐ prewes   V. ad 176.
ⁿ eerys. Ears *for the* pots V. 185.
ᵒ rofys   rofes
ᵖ ſtele.   ſtalks.
ᑫ þ̃. there, ɪ. e where. V 170.

Sacchus.

[ 81 ]

### Sachus <sup>r</sup>.     XX. VIII. XVIII.

Take smale Sachellis of canuas and fille hem full of þ same fars <sup>s</sup> ⁊ seeþ hē. and whan þey buth ynowʒ take of the canvas. rost hem ⁊ colō hem ⁊c.

### Burſews <sup>t</sup>.     XX VIII. XIX.

Take Pork. seeþ it and grynde it smale wiþ sodden ayren. do þ<sup>r</sup>to gode powdōs and hole spices and salt w<sup>t</sup> sug. make þ<sup>r</sup>of smale ballꝭ, and cast hē in a batō <sup>u</sup> of ayren. ⁊ wete hē in flo͞. and frye hē in grece as frytōs <sup>x</sup>. and sue hem forth.

### Spynoch <sup>y</sup> yfryed.     XX IX.

Take Spynoch. p̄boile hē ī seþyng wat̄. take hē up and p̄ſſe ... cut of þ wat̄ <sup>z</sup> and hem <sup>a</sup> ī two. frye hē ī oile clene. ⁊ do þ<sup>r</sup>to powdō. ⁊ sue forth.

---

<sup>r</sup> Sachus. I suppose *sacks.*

<sup>s</sup> same fars. viz as 174

<sup>t</sup> Bursews. Different from *Bursen* in Nº 11, therefore qu. etymon

<sup>u</sup> Batō batter.

<sup>x</sup> frytōs. fritters.

<sup>y</sup> Spynoches. Spinage, which we use in the singular

<sup>z</sup> out of the water. dele *of*, or it may mean, *when cut of the water.*

<sup>a</sup> hem r. *hexe.*

L          Benes

### Benes yfryed. XX IX. I.

Take benes and seeþ hē almost til þey bersten. take and wryng out þ wat clene. do þto Oynons yſode and ymynced. and garlec pw. frye hem ĩ oile. oþ ĩ grece. & do þto powdo douce. & ſūe it forth.

### Ryſhews [b] of Fruyt. XX IX II.

Take Fyg and raiſons. pyke hē and walſshe hē in Wyne. grynde hē wiþ apples and peer ypared and ypiked clene. do þto gode powdos. and hole ſpices. make ball þof. fryē ĩ oile and ſūe hē forth.

### Daryols [c]. XX IX III.

Take Creme of Cowe mylke. oþ of Almand. do þto ayren w ſug, ſafron, and ſalt. medle it yfere. do it ĩ a coffyn. of II. ynche depe. bake it wel and ſūe it forth.

### Flaumpeyns [d]. XX IX IIII.

Take fat Pork yſode. pyke it clene. grynde it ſmale. grynde Cheſe & do þto. wiþ ſug and gode powdos.

---

[b] Ryſhews *ryſchewſes*, Contents. Qu.
[c] Daryols. Qu.
[d] Flaumpeyns. *Flaumpens*, Contents. V. Nº 113.

make

make a coffyn of an ynche depe. and do þis fars þin. make a thynne foile of gode paſt ꝛ kerue out þoff ſmale poyntꝭ ͤ. frye hī in fars ᶠ. ꝛ bake it up ꝛc.

### Chewetꝭ ᵍ on Fleſhe Day.     xx ix. v.

Take þ lire of Pork and kerue it al to pecys. and henñ þwith and do it ī a panne and frye it ꝛ make a Coffyn as to ʰ a pye ſmale ꝛ do þinne. ꝛ do ſuppon ʒolk of ayreñ. harde. powdo of gyng and ſalt, coue it ꝛ fry it ī grece. oþ bake it wel and ſue it forth.

### Chewet on Fyſsh Day.     xx ix. vi.

Take Turbut. haddok. Codlyng. and hake. and ſeeþ it. grynde it ſmale. and do þto Datꝭ. ygronden. rayſons pyn. gode powdo and ſalt. make a Coffyn as tofore ſaide. cloſe þis þin. and frye it ī oile. oþ ſtue it in gyng ſug. oþ ī wyne. oþ bake it. ꝛ ſue forth.

### Haſtletꝭ ⁱ of Fruyt.     xx ix. vii.

Take Fyg iqrterid ᵏ, Rayſons hool datꝭ and Almandꝭ

---

ᵉ Points, ſeems the ſame as *Prews*, N° 176.

ᶠ in fars, f. *in the jars*, and yet the Fars is diſpoſed of before; ergo quære.

ᵍ Chewets V. 186.     ʰ as to, as for. V. N° 177.

ⁱ Haſtletes. *Haſteletes*, Contents.

ᵏ iqrterid. iquartcred.

hoole. and ryne¹ hē on a fpyt and rooft hē. and eᵑ-
doreᵐ hem as pōme dorryes ⁊ ſūe hē forth.

### Comadoreⁿ. XX IX. VII.

Take Fẙg and Raiſoñs. pyke hem and waiſhe hē
clene. ſkalde hē ĩ wyne. grynde hē right ſmale. caſt
ſuͬg ĩ þ ſelf wyne. and foñde it togẙd. drawe it up
thᵤrgh a ſtẙnȯ. ⁊ alye up þ fruẙt þͨw. take gode
peervs and Applͬ pare hem and take þ beſt, grynde
hem ſmale and caſt ͬþto. ſet a pot on þͨ fuẙrᵒ wiþ
oẙle and caſt alle þiſe þẙng þinne. and ſtere it warliche,
and kepe it wel fro breͨnyng. and whan it is fyned
caſt ͬþto powdͬͦs of gẙng of canel. of galyngale. hool
cloẇ fͦ ot canel. ⁊ macẙs hoole. caſt þto pyn̄ a litel
frẙed ĩ oile ⁊ ſalt, and whan it is ynowȝ fyned⸝ take
it up and do it ĩ a veſſel ⁊ lat it kele. and whan it is
colde⸝ kerue out w a knyf ſmale pecys of þͨ gretneſſe
⁊ of þͨ length of a litel fẙng. ⁊ cloſe it faſt ĩ gode
paſt. ⁊ frye hē ĩ oile. ⁊ ſūe forth.

¹ ryne    run.
ᵐ endore    endorſe, MS. Ed. 42. II. 6. v. ad 147.
ⁿ Comadore    Qu.
ᵒ Fuẙr    ᵢie.

Chaſtletͬ

[ 85 ]

Chastlet ᵖ.   XX IX. IX.

Take and make a foyle of gode past with a roller of a foot brode. ⁊ lyng ᵠ by cūpas. make iiii Coffyns of þ self past uppon þ roller þ gretnesse of þ smale of þyn Arme. of vi ynche depnesse. make þ gretust ʳ ĩ þ myddell. fasten þ foile ĩ þ mouth upwarde. ⁊ fasten þee ˢ oþe foure ĩ euy syde. kerūe out keyntlich kyrnels ᵗ above ĩ þ mane of bataiwyng ᵘ and drye hē harde ĩ an Ovene. oþ ĩ þ Sūne. In þ myddel Coffyn do a fars of Pork w gode Pork ⁊ ayren rawe wiþ salt. ⁊ colō it wiþ safron and do in anoþ Creme of Almand. and helde ˣ it in anoþ ʸ creme of Cowe mylke w ayren. colō it w sandr. anoþ man. Fars of Fyg. of raysons. of Apples. of Peer. ⁊ holde it in bron ᶻ. anoþ

---

ᵖ Chastelets. Little castles, as is evident from the kernelling and the battlements mentioned *Castles of jelly templewise made*. Lel. Coll IV. p. 227.

ᵠ lyng   longer.

ʳ gretust. greatest.

ˢ þee, i e thou.

ᵗ kyrnels. Battlements. V. Gloss Keyntlich, quaintly, curiously. V. Gloss.

ᵘ bataiwyng. embattelling.

ˣ helde. put, cast

ʸ another. As the middle one and only two more are provided for, the two remaining were to be filled, I presume, in the same manner alternately.

ᶻ holde it bron. make it brown.

mane.

[ 86 ]

mane. do fars as to frytos blanched. and colo͝ it with
grene. put þis to þ ovene ⁊ bake it wel. ⁊ sue it forth
w ew ardant ᵃ.

For to make II.ᵇ pecys of Flefsh  
    to faften togy͝d.     xx IX. X.

Take a pece of frefsh Flefh and do it ĩ a pot for to
feeþ. or take a pece of frefsh Flefsh and kerue it al
to gobet. do it ĩ a pot to feeþ. ⁊ take þ wofe ᶜ of
comfery ⁊ put it ĩ þ pot to þ flefsh ⁊ it fhal faftẽ and,
⁊ fo sue it forth.

Pur fait Ypocras ᵈ.    xx IX. XI.

Treys Unces de canell. ⁊ iij unces de gyngen.
fpykenard de Spayn le pays dun dener ᵉ. garyngale ᶠ.
clowes, gylofre. pocur long ᵍ, noiez mugadez ʰ. ma-

---

ᵃ ew ardant. hot water. *Eau*, water, anciently written *eue*.

ᵇ .II. *Two*, Contents

ᶜ wofe Roots of comfrey are of a very glutinous nature Quincy, Difpenf p 100 *Wofe* is A S *pey*, *humour*, juice. See J—s, v. *Wo*, and Mr Strype's Life of Stow, p VIII.

ᵈ Pur fait Ypocras. Id eft, *Pour faire Ypocras*, a whole pipe of which was provided for archbifhop Nevill's feaft about A D. 1466. So that it was in vaft requeft formerly.

ᵉ = pays d'un dener, i e *le pays d'un Dener*.

ᶠ garyngale, i e. *galingale*.

ᵍ pocur long, r pour long, i e *poure long*.

ʰ mugadez, r mufadez, but q as the French is *muguette* Nutmegs.

ziozame

ziozame ͥ cardemonij ᵏ de chefcuñ 1. q̃rt' douce ˡ grayne
⁊ ᵐ de paradys flo̊ de queynel ⁿ de chefcuñ dĩ ᵒ unce de
tout. foit fait powdo̊ ⁊c.

For to make blank mang ᵖ. IX XII.

Put Rys ĩ wat̃ al a nyzt and at morowe waifshe h̃e
clene. aftward put h̃e to þ fyr̃ fort ᑫ þ þey berft ⁊ not
to myche. ffithen ʳ take brawn of Capons, or of henn.
foden ⁊ drawe ˢ it fmale. aft̃ take mylke of Almand.
and put ĩ to þ Ryys ⁊ boile it. and whan it is yboiled
put ĩ þ brawn ⁊ alye it þwith. þ it be wel chargeant ᵗ
and mung it fynelich ᵘ wel þ it fit not ˣ to þ pot. and
whan it is ynowʒ ⁊ chargeant. do þto fug gode part,
put þin almand. fryed ĩ white grece. ⁊ dreffe it forth.

ͥ maziozame, r. marjorame

ᵏ Cardemonij, r. *Cardamoaes*.

ˡ 1 qrtdouce, r. *d'once*. Five penny weights.

ᵐ ⁊ dele.

ⁿ queynel  Perhaps *Canell*, but qu. as that is named before.

ᵒ dj̃. dimid.

ᵖ blank mang  Very different from that we make now. V. 36.

ᑫ fyr̃ fort. ftrong fire.

ʳ ffithen. then.

ˢ drawe. make.

ᵗ chargeant. ftiff. So below, *ynowhz & chargeant* V 193, 194. V Gloff.

ᵘ mung it fynelich ʳ wel. ftir it very well

ˣ fit not.  adheres not, and thereby burns not. Ufed now in the North.

For

[ 88 ]

For to make blank Defne ⱽ.  XX IX. XIIIᵈ

Take Brawn of Henn̄ or of Capon̄s yſoden withoute þe ſkyn. ꝫ hewe hē as ſmale as þ may. ꝫ gnde hem ī a morṫ. afṫ take gode mylke of Almand ꝫ put þe brawn þin. ꝫ ſtere it wel togyd ꝫ do hem to ſeeþ. ꝫ take flo of Rys ꝫ amydōn ꝫ alay it. ſo þat it be chargeant. ꝫ do þto ſug a gode pty. ꝫ a pty of white grece. and when it is put ī diſh ſtrewe uppon it blan̄che powdo. and þen̄ne put in blank deſire and mawmenye ᶻ ī diſhes togider. and ſūe forth.

For to make Mawmenny ᵃ.  XX IX. XIIII.

Take þe cheſe and of Fleſh of Capon̄s or of Henn̄. ꝫ hakke ſmale in a morṫ. take mylke of Almand w þe broth oþ freiſh Beef, oþ freſh fleſh. ꝫ put the fleſh ī þe mylke oþ in the broth and ſet hē to þ frye ᵇ. ꝫ alye hē up w flo of Ryſe. or gaſtbon ᶜ. or amydōn. as chargeant as þ blanke deſire. ꝫ w zolk of ayren and

---

ᵛ blank *Defve. Dfire*, Contents; recṫè. V. Gloſſ. The Recipe in MS Ed 29 is much the ſame with this.

ᶻ Mawmenye See Nᵒ 194.

ᵃ Mawmenny *Mawmoure*, Contents *Mawrene*, MS. Ed 29, 30 vide Nᵒ 193. See Preface for a facſimile of this Recipe.

ᵇ þ frye. an f.re?

ᶜ gaſtbon. Q !.

I fuſion

ſafroñ for to make it zelow. and when it is dreſſit in diſsh w blank deſir ſtyk above clow de gilofre. ⁊ ſtrewe Powdo of galyngale above. and ſue it forth.

### The Pety Puant [d]. XX IX. XV.

Take male Marow [e]. hole parade [f] and kerue it rawe. powdo of Gyng. zolk of Ayreñ, dat mynced. raiſoñs of corañce. ſalt a lytel. ⁊ loke þ þ make þy paſt with zolkes of Ayren. ⁊ þat no wat come þto. and foṁe þy coffyn. and make up þy paſt.

### Payn puff [g]. XX. IX. XVI.

Eodem ṁ fait payn puff. but make it more tendre þ paſt. and loke þ paſt be roñde of þ payn puf as a coffyn ⁊ a pye.

## [h] rplicit.

[d] pety puant. a paſte, therefore, perhaps, *paty*, but qu. the latter word

[e] male Marow. Qu.

[f] parade Qu.

[g] Payn puff. Contents has, *And the pete puant*

[h] A blank was left in the original for a large *F*.

[ 90 ]

## The following Memorandum at the End of the Roll.

" Antiquum hoc monumentum oblatum et miffum eft majeftati veftræ vicefimo feptimo die menfis Julij, anno regno veftri fæliciffimi vicefimo vuj ab humilimo veftro fubdito, veftræq majeftati fideliffimo

E<sup>D</sup> STAFFORD,
Hæres domus fubverfæ Buckinghamienf."

N.B. He was Lord Stafford and called Edward.

Edw. D. of Bucks beheaded 1521. 13 H. VIII.
|
Henry, reftored in blood by H. VIII.; and again
| [1 Ed. VI.
Edw. aged 21, 1592; born 1592. 21. ob. 1525.
| 21 [f. 1625.
Edw. b. 1600. ———
1571 born.

# ANCIENT COOKERY.

## A. D. 1381.

*Hic incipiunt universa servicia tam de carnibus quam de piffibus*[a].

### I. For to make Furmenty [a].

NYM clene Wete and bray it in a morter wel that the holys [b] gon al of and feyt [c] yt til it brefte and nym yt up. and lat it kele [d] and nym fayre frefch broth and fwete mylk of Almandys or fwete mylk of kyne and temper yt al. and nym the yolkys of eyryn [e]. boyle it a lityl and fet yt adōn and meffe yt forthe wyth fat venyfon and frefh moton.

---

[a] See again, Nº I. of the fecond part of this treatife.
[b] Hulls.
[c] Mifwritten for *feyth* or *fethe*, i. e. feeth.
[d] cool
[e] eggs.

II. For to make Pise of Almayne.

Nym wyte Pisyn and wasch hem and seth hem a good wyle sithsyn wasch hem in golde [f] watyr unto the holys gon of alle in a pot and kever it wel that no breth passe owt and boyle hem ryzt wel and do therto god mylk of Almandys and a party of flowr of ris and salt and safron and messe yt forthe.

III.

Cranys and Herons schulle be euarūd [g] wyth Lardons of swyne and rostyd and etyn wyth gyngynyr.

IV.

Pecokys and Partrigchis schul ben yparboyld and lardyd and etyn wyth gyngenyr.

V. Morterelys [h].

Nym hennyn and porke and seth hem togedere nym the lyre [i] of the hennyn and the porke and hakkyth smale and grynd hit al to dust and wyte bred therwyth and temper it wyth the selve broth and wyth heyryn and colure it with safron and boyle it and disch it and cast theron powder of peper and of gyngynyr and serve it forthe.

---

[f] cold

[g] Perhaps *enarm'd* or *enarned*. See Mr. Bruder's Roll, N° 146

[h] V Mortrews in Gloss.    [i] Flesh.

## VI. Caponys in concys.

Schal be fodyn. Nym the lyre and brek it fmal in a morter and peper and wyte bred therwyth and temper it wyth ale and ley it wyth the capon Nym hard fodyn eyryn and hewe the wyte fmal and kafte thereto and nym the zolkys al hole and do hem in a dyfch and boyle the capon and colowre it wyth fafron and falt it and meffe it forthe.

## VII. Hennys[k] in bruet.

Schullyn be fcaldyd and fodyn wyth porke and grynd pepyr and comyn bred and ale and temper it wyth the felve broth and boyle and colowre it wyth fafron and falt it and meffe it forthe.

## VIII. Harys[l] in cmee[m].

Schul be parboylyd and lardyd and roftid and nym onyons and myce hem rizt fmal and fry hem in wyte gres and grynd peper bred and ale and the onions therto and coloure it wyth fafron and falt it and ferve it forth.

## IX. Haris in Talbotays.

Schul be hewe in gobbettys and fodyn with al the blod Nym bred piper and ale and grynd togedere

---

[k] Hens.      [l] Hares.
[m] Perhaps *Cinee*, for fee N° 51.

and

and temper it with the felve broth and boyle it and falt it and ferve it forthe.

### X. Conynggys [n] in Gravey.

Schul be fodyn and hakkyd in gobbettys and grynd gyngynyr galyngale and canel and temper it up with god almand mylk and boyle it and nym macys and clowys and keft [o] therin and the conynggis alfo and falt hym [p] and ferve it forthe.

### XI. For to make a Colys [q].

Nym hennys and fchald hem wel. and feth hem after and nym the lyre and hak yt fmal and bray it with otyn grotys in a morter and with wyte bred and temper it up wyth the broth Nym the grete bonys and grynd hem al to duft and keft hem al in the broth and mak it thorw a clothe and boyle it and ferve it forthe.

### XII. For to make Nombles [r].

Nym the nomblys of the venyfon and wafch hem clene in water and falt hem and feth hem in tweye waterys grynd pepyr bred and ale and temper it wyth the fecunde brothe and boyle it and hak the nomblys and do theryn and ferve it forthe.

[n] Rabbits
[o] .t, or perhaps lt.
[r] Umbles.
[p] Caft
[q] Cullis. V. Preface.

[ 95 ]

XIII. For to make blanche Brewet de Alyngyn.

Nym kedys [s] and chekenys and hew hem in morsellys and feth hem in almand mylk or in kyne mylke grynd gyngyner galingale and caft therto and boyle it and ferve it forthe.

XIV. For to make Blomanger [t].

Nym rys and lefe hem and wafch hem clene and do thereto god almande mylk and feth hem tyl they al to breft and than lat hem kele and nym the lyre of the hennyn or of capons and grynd hem fmal keft therto wite grefe and boyle it Nym blanchyd almandys and fafron and fet hem above in the dyfche and ferve yt forthe.

XV. For to make Afronchemoyle [u].

Nym eyren wyth al the wyte and myfe bred and fchepys [w] talwe as gret as dyfes [x] grynd peper and fafron and caft therto and do hit in the fchepis wombe feth it wel and dreffe it forthe of brode leches thynne.

---

[s] Kids.

[t] Blanc-manger. See again, N° 33, 34. II. N° 7. Chauc writes it *Blankmanger*.

[u] Frenchemulle d'un mouton. A fheeps call, or kell. Cotgra\ Junius, v. *Moil*, fays, "a French moile Chaucero eft cibus deli\ " tior, a difh made of marrow and grated bread."

[w] Sheep's fat.

[x] dice, fquare bits, or bits as big as dice.

[ 96 ]

### XVI. For to make Brymeus.

Nym the tharmys ʸ of a pygge and wafch hem clene in water and falt and feth hem wel and than hak hem fmale and grynd pepyr and fafron bred and ale and boyle togedere Nym wytys of eyryn and knede it wyth flour and mak fmal pelotys ᶻ and fry hem with wyte grees and do hem in difches above that othere mete and ferve it forthe.

### XVII. For to make Appulmos ᵃ.

Nym appelyn and feth hem and lat hem kele and make hem thorw a clothe and on flefch dayes kaft therto god fat breyt ᵇ of Bef and god wyte grees and fugar and fafron and almande mylk on fyfch dayes oyle de olyve and gode powdres ᶜ and ferve it forthe.

### XVIII. For to make a Froys ᵈ.

Nym Veel and feth it wel and hak it fmal and grynd bred peper and fafron and do thereto and frye yt and preffe it wel upon a bord and dreffe yt forthe.

---

ʸ Rops, guts, puddings.
ᶻ Balls, pellets, from the French *pelote*.
ᵃ See Nº 35
ᵇ Breth, i. e. broth See Nº 58.
ᶜ Spices ground fmall. See Nº 27, 28. 35. 58. II. Nº 4. 17. or perhaps of Galingale. II. 20. 24.
ᵈ a Fraife.

XIX.

### XIX. For to make Fruturs [e].

Nym flowre and eyryn and grynd peper and safron and mak therto a batour and par aplyn and kyt hem to brode penys [f] and kest hem theryn and fry hem in the batour wyth fresch grees and serve it forthe.

### XX. For to make chanke [g].

Nym Porke and seth it wel and hak yt smal nym eyryn wyth al the wytys and swyng hem wel al togedere and kast god swete mylke thereto and boyle yt and messe it forthe.

### XXI. For to make Juffel.

Nym eyryn wyth al the wytys and mice bred grynd pepyr and safron and do therto and temper yt wyth god fresch broth of porke and boyle it wel and messe yt forthe.

### XXII. For to make Gees [h] in ochepot [i].

Nym and schald hem wel and hew hem wel in gobettys al rawe and seth hem in her owyn grees and cast therto wyn or ale a cuppe ful and myce onyons smal and do therto and boyle yt and salt yt and messe yt forthe.

---

[e] Fritters.    [f] Pieces as bread in pennies, or perhaps pence.
[g] Quære    Ge .
[i] Hochepot. Vide Gloss.

XXIII For to make eyryn in bruet.

Nym water and welle ᵏ yt and brek eyryn and kaſt ther in and grind peper and ſafron and temper up wyth ſwete mylk and boyle it and hakke cheſe ſmal and caſt therin and meſſe yt forthe.

XXIV. For to make crayton [1].

Tak chec nys nd ſchald hem and ſeth hem and grynd zyngen' other pepyr and comyn and temper it up wyt god mylk and do the checonys theryn and boyle hem and ſerve yt forthe.

XXV. For to make mylk roſt.

Nym ſwete mylk and do yt in a panne nyn ᵐ eyryn wyth al e wyte and ſwyng hem wel and caſt therto and colour it wyth ſafron and boyl it tyl yt wexe thykke and tharne ſeth ⁿ yt thorw a culdore ᵒ and nym that leyt ᵖ and preſſe yt up on a bord and wan yt ys cold larde it ard ſcher yt on ſchyverys and roſte yt on a grydern and ſerve yt forthe.

---

ᵏ Quære the meaning
[1] Vide ad Nᵒ 60 of the Roll.
ᵐ Read *nym*.
ⁿ ſtrain See Nᵒ 27.
ᵒ Culander
ᵖ That which is left in the cullinder.

XXVI. For to make cryppys [q].

Nym flour and wytys of eyryn fugur other hony and fweyng togedere and mak a batour nym wyte grees and do yt in a pofnet and caft the batur thereyn and ftury to thou have many [r] and tak hem up and meffe hem wyth the frutours and ferve forthe.

XXVII. For to make Berandyles [s].

Nym Hennys and feth hem wyth god Buf and wan hi ben fodyn nym the Hennyn and do awey the bonys and bray fmal yn a moiter and temper yt wyth the broth and feth yt thorw a culdore and caft therto powder of gyngenyr and fugur and graynys of powmis gernatys [t] and boyle yt and dreffe yt in dyfches and caft above clowvs gylofres [u] and maces and god powder [x] ferve yt forthe.

XXVIII. For to make capons in caffelys.

Nym caponys and fchald hem nym a penne and opyn the fkyn at the hevyd [y] and blowe hem tyl the fkyn ryfe from the flefshe and do of the fkyn al hole

---

[q] Meaning, *crifps*. V. Gloff.
[r] It will run into lumps, I fuppofe.
[s] Quære the meaning
[t] Pomegranates. V N° 39.
[u] Not clove-gilliflowers, but *cloves*. See N° 30, 31, 40.
[x] See N° 17, note [c].
[y] Head. Sax. heopob and hevob, hence our *Head*.

and feth the lyre of Hennyn and zolkys of heyryn and god powder and make a Farfure [z] and fil ful the fkyn and parboyle yt and do yt on a fpete and roft yt and droppe [a] yt wyth zolkys of eyryn and god powder roftyng and nym the caponys body and larde yt and rofte it and nym almaunde mylk and amydon [b] and mak a batur and droppe the body roftyng and ferve yt forthe.

XXX. For to make the blank furry [c].

Tak brann [d] of caponys other of hennys and the thyes [e] wythowte the fkyn and kerf hem fmal als thou mayft and grynd hem fmal in a morter and tak mylk of Almaundys and do yn the branne and grynd hem thanne togedere and and feth hem togeder' and tak flour of rys other amydon and lye it that yt be charchant and do therto fugur a god parti and a party of wyt grees and boyle yt and wan yt ys don in dyfchis ftraw upon blank poudere and do togedere blank de fury and manmene [f] in a dyfch and ferve it forthe.

---

[z] ftuffing.
[a] bafte
[b] Vide Gloff.
[c] Vide *Blank Defire* in Gloff.
[d] Perhaps *brawn*, the brawny part. See N° 33. and the Gloff.
[e] Thighs.
[f] See the next number. Quære *Maumeny*.

XXX. For to make manmene ᵍ.

Tak the thyys ʰ other the flefch of the caponys fede ⁱ hem and kerf hem fmal into a morter and tak mylk of Almandys wyth broth of frefch Buf and do the flefch in the mylk or in the broth and do yt to the fyre and myng yt togedere wyth flour of Rys othere of waftelys als charchaut als the blank de fure and wyth the zolkys of eyryn for to make it zelow and fafron and wan yt ys dieffyd in dyfches wyth blank de fure ftraw upon clowys of gelofie ᵏ and ftraw upon powdre of galentyn and ferve yt forthe.

XXXI. For to make Bruet of Almayne.

Tak Partrichys roftyd and checonys and qualys roftyd and larkys ywol and demembre the other and mak a god cawdel and dreffe the flefch in a dyfch and ftrawe powder of galentyn therupon. ftyk upon clowys of gelofre and ferve yt forthe.

XXXII. For ro make Bruet of Lombardye.

Tak chekenys or hennys or othere flefch and mak the colowre als red as any blod and tak peper and kanel and gyngyner bied ˡ and grynd hem in a morter

---

ᵍ Vide Number 29, and the Gloff.

ʰ Thighs.

ⁱ Quære

ᵏ See Nº 27, note ᵘ.

ˡ This is ftill in ufe, and, it feems, is an old compound.

and

and a porcōn of bred and mak that bruer thenne and do that flefch in that broth and mak hem boyle togedere and ftury it wel and tak eggys and temper hem wyth Jus of Parcyle and wryng hem thorwe a cloth and wan that bruet is boylyd do that therto and meng tham togedere wyth fayr grees fo that yt be fat ynow and ferve yt forthe.

XXXIII. For to make Blomanger [m].

Do Ris in water al nyzt and upon the morwe wafch hem wel and do hem upon the fyre for to [n] they breke and nozt for to muche and tak Brann [o] of Caponis fodyn and wel ydraw [p] and fmal and tak almaund mylk and boyle it wel wyth ris and wan it is yboylyd do the flefch therin fo that it be charghaunt and do therto a god party of fugure and wan it ys dreffyd forth in difchis ftraw theron blaunche Pouder and ftrik [q] theron Almaundys fryed wyt wyte grece [r] and ferve yt forthe.

XXXIV. For to make Sandale that party to Blomanger.

Tak Flefch of Caponys and of Pork fodyn kerf yt fmal into a morter togedere and bray that wel. and

---

[m] See Nº 14.
[n] till. *for*, however, abounds.
[o] See Nº 29 note [d]
[p] Perhap., *ftrained*. See Nº 49, and Part II. Nº 33.
[q] Perhaps, *ftik*, i. e. ftick, but fee 34.
[r] Grefe. Fat, or lard.

temper

temper it up wyth broth of Caponys and of Pork that yt be wel charchaunt alfo the crem of Almaundys and grynd egg⁹ and fafron or fandies togedere that it be coloured and ftraw upon Powder of Galentyn and ftrik thereon clowys and maces and ferve it forthe.

### XXXV. For to make Apulmos ˢ.

Tak Applys and feth hem and let hem kele and after mak hem thorwe a cloth and do hem in a pot and kaft to that mylk of Almaundys wyth god broth of Buf in Flefch dayes do bred ymved ᵗ therto. And the fifch dayes do therto oyle of olyve and do therto fugur and colour it wyth fafron and ftrew theron Powder and ferve it forthe.

### XXXVI. For to make mete Gelee ᵘ that it be wel chariaunt.

Tak wyte wyn and a party of water and fafron and gode fpicis and flefch of Piggys or of Hennys or frefch Fifch and boyle them togedere and after wan yt ys boylyd and cold dres yt in difchis and ferve yt forthe.

---

ˢ See Nº 17.
ᵗ f. ymyced, i. e. *minced.*
ᵘ meat jelly.

## XXXVII. For to make Murrey [x].

Tak mulbery [y] and bray hem in a morter and wpyng [z] hem thorth a cloth and do hem in a pot over the fyre and do ther'to fat bred and wyte greffe and let it nazt boyle no ofter than onys and do ther'to a god party of fugur and zif yt be nozt ynowe colowrd brey mulburus and ferve yt forthe.

## XXXVIII. For to make a penche of Egges.

Tak water and do it in a panne to the fyre and lat yt fethe and after tak eggs and brek hem and caft hem in the water and after tak a chefe and kerf yt on fowr paruns and caft in the water and wanne the chefe and the eggys ben wel fodyn tak hem owt of the water and wafch hem in clene water and tak waftel breed and temper yt wyth mylk of a kow. and after do yt over the fyre and after forfy yt wyth gyngener and ryth comyn and colowr yt wyth faf-ron and lye yt wyth eggys and oyle the fewe wyth Boter and kep wel the chefe owt and dreffe the fewe and d mo [a] eggys ther'on al ful and kerf thy chefe in lytyl fchyms and do hem in the fewe wyth eggys and ferve yt forthe.

---

[x] Morrey Part II N° 26

[y] This is to be underftood plurali, *quafi* mulberries.

[z] Read wryng. For fee part II. N° 17. 28. Chaucer, v. *wronge* and *wrng*

[a] Perhaps, *do mo*, i. e. put more.

## XXXIX. For to make Comyn.

Tak god Almaunde mylk and lat yt boyle and do ther'in amydoñ wyth flowr of Rys and colowr yt wyth fafroñ and after dreffe yt wyth graynis of Poungarnetts [b] other wyth reyfens zyf thow haft non other and tak fugur and do theryn and ferve it forthe.

## XIV. For to make Fruturs [c].

Tak crommys [d] of wyte bred and the flowris of the fwete Appyltre and zolkys of Eggys and bray hem togedere in a morter and temper yt up wyth wyte wyn and mak yt to fethe and wan yt is thykke do thereto god fpicis of gyngener galyngale canel and clowys gelofie and ferve yt forth.

## XLI. For to make Rofee [e].

Tak the flowris of Rofys and wafch hem wel in water and after bray hem wel in a morter and than tak Almondys and temper hem and feth hem and after tak flefch of capons or of hennys and hac yt fmale and than bray hem wel in a morter and than do yt in the Rofe [f] fo that the flefch acorde wyth the mylk and fo that the mete be charchaunt and after do yt to the fyre to boyle and do thereto fugur and fafroñ

---

[b] Vide N° 27.
[d] Crumbs.
[f] i. e. Rofee.

[c] Fritters.
[e] V. de N° 47.

that yt be wel ycolowrd and rofy of levys and of the forſeyde flowrys and ſerve yt forth.

XLII. For to make Pommedorry [g].

Tak Buf and hewe yt ſmal al raw and caſt yt in a morter and grynd yt nozt to ſmal tak ſafron and grynd ther'wyth wan yt ys grounde tak the wyte of the eyryn zyf yt be nozt ſtyf. Caſt into the Buf pouder of Pepyr olde reſyns and of coronſe ſet over a panne wyth fayr water and mak pelotys of the Buf and wan the water and the pelots ys wel yboylyd and [h] ſet yt adon and kele yt and put yt on a broche and roſt yt and endorre yt wyth zolkys of eyryn and ſerve yt forthe.

XLIII. For to make Longe de Buf [i].

Nym the tonge of the rether [k] and ſchalde and ſchawe [l] yt wel and rizt clene and feth yt and ſethe nym a broche [m] and larde yt wyth lardons and wyth clowys and gelofr' and do it roſtyng and drop yt wel yt roſtyd [n] wyth zolkys of eyrin and dreſſe it forthe.

[g] Vide N° 58.
[h] dele *and*
[i] Neat's Tongue. *Make* ſignifies *to dreſs*, as II 12.
[k] The ox or cow. Lye in Jun. Etymolog. v. *Rother*.
[l] Shave, ſcrape.
[m] A larding-pin.
[n] Pehaps, *uyk it roſtyth*.

XLIV.

### XLIV. For to make Rew de Rumfy.

Nym fwynys fet and eyr º and make hem clene and feth hem alf wyth wyn and half wyth water caft mycyd onyons ther'to and god fpicis and wan they be yfodyn nym and rofty hem in a gryder' wan it is yroftyd keft thereto of the felve broth by lyed wyth amydon and anyeyd onyons ᴾ and ferve yt forth.

### XLV. For to make Bukkenade ᵠ.

Nym god frefch flefch wat maner fo yt be and hew yt in fmale morfelys and feth yt wyth gode frefch buf and caft ther'to gode mynced onyons and gode fpiceiye and alyth ʳ wyth eyryn and boyle and dreffe yt forth.

### XLVI. For to make fpine ˢ.

Nym the flowrys of the haw thorn clene gaderyd and bray hem al to duft and temper hem wyth Almaunde mylk and aly yt wyth amydon and wyth eyryn wel pykke ᵗ and boyle it and meffe yt forth and flowrys and levys abovy on ᵘ.

---

º To be underftood plurally, *Ears.*

ᴾ Mifwritten for *mycyd,* i. e. minced onyons.

ᵠ Vide Nº 52.

ʳ Stiffen, thicken it See Nº 44. where *lyed* has that fenfe See alfo 46.

ˢ This difh, no doubt, takes its name from *Spina,* of which it is made.

ᵗ Read, þykke, *thykke.*

ᵘ It means *laid upon it.*

[ 108 ]

XLVII. For to make Rosee [x] and Frese and Swan schal be ymad in the selve maner.

Nym pyggus and hennys and other maner fresch flesch and hew yt in morselys and seth yt in wyth wyn' and ' gyngyner and galyngale and gelofr' and canel [z] and bray yt wel and kest thereto and alye yt wyth amydon other wyth flowr of rys.

XLVIII. For to make an amendement Formete that ys to [a] salt and over mychyl.

Nym etemele and bynd yt in a fayr lynnen clowt and lat yt horge in the pot so that yt thowche nozt the bottym and lat it hongy ther'ynne a god wyle and seþh [b] set yt fro the fyre and let yt kele and yt schal be fresch ynow wythoute any other maner licowr ydo ther'to.

XLIX. For to make Rapy [c].

Tak Fygys and reysyns and wyn and grynd hem togeder tak and draw hem thorw a cloth and do ther'to powder of Alkenet other of rys and do ther'to a god quantite of pepir and vyneger and boyle it togeder and messe yt and serve yt forth.

[x] Vide N° 41.
[y] Perhaps, *u = yn crub.*
[z] Cinamon Vide Gloss.
[a] ic ei, *too.*
[b] Read, *seþb*, i. e. then
[c] Vide Part II. N° 1. 28.

L. For

### L. For to make an Egge Dows [d].

Tak Almaundys and mak god mylk and temper wyth god wyneger clene tak reyſynys and boyle hem in clene water and tak the reyſynıs and tak hem owt of the water and boyle hem wyth mylk and zyf thow wyl colowr yt wyth ſafroñ and ſerve yt forth.

### LI. For to make a mallard in cyney [e].

Tak a mallard and pul hym drye and ſwyng over the fyre draw hym but lat hym touche no water and hew hym ın gobettys and do hym ın a pot of clene water boyle hem wel and tak onyons and boyle and bred and pepyr and grynd togedere and draw thorw a cloth temper wyth wyn and boyle yt and ſerve yt forth.

### LII. For to make a Bukkenade [f].

Tak veel and boyle ıt tak zolkys of eggys and mak hem thykke tak macıs and powdr' of gyngyn' and powder of peper and boyle yt togeder and meſſe yt forth.

---

[d] Vide ad Part II Nº 21. There are no eggs concerned, ſo no doubt ıt ſhould be *Eger Dows*. Vide Gloſſ.

[e] See Nº 8.

[f] Vide Nº 45.

## LIII. For to make a Roo Broth [g].

Tak Parſile and Yſop and Sauge and hak yt ſmal boil it in wyn and in water and a lytyl powdr' of peper and meſſe yt forth.

## LIV. For to mak a Bruet of Sarcyneſſe.

Tak the lyre of the freſch Buf and bet it al in pecis and bred and fry yt in freſch gres tak it up and and drye it and do yt in a veſſel wyth wyn and ſugur and powdr' of clowys boyle yt togedere tyl the fleſch have drong the liycour' and take the almande mylk and quibibz macis and clowys and boyle hem togeder tak the fleſch and do ther'to and meſſe it forth.

## LV. For to make a Gely [h].

Tak hoggys fet other pyggys other erys other partrichys other chiconys and do hem togeder' and ſeþh [i] hem in a pot and do hem in flowr' of canel and clowys other or grounde [k] do ther'to vineger and tak and do the broth in a clene veſſel of al thys and tak the Fleſch and kerf yt in ſmal morſelys and do yt therein

---

[g] *Deer* or *Roes* are not mentioned, as in Mr Brander's Roll, Nº 14, ergo quære. It is a meager buſineſs. Can it mean *Rue-Broth* for penitents?

[h] Jelly.

[i] ſeþ, i. e. ſeeth.

[k] Not clearly expreſſed. It means either Cinamon or Cloves, and either in flour or ground.

tak

tak powder of galyngale and caſt above and lat yt kels tak bronches of the lorer tr' and ſtyk over it and kep yt al ſo longe as thou wilt and ſerve yt forth.

LVI. For to kepe Veniſon fro reſtyng.

Tak veniſon wan yt ys newe and cuver it haſtely wyth Fern that no wynd may come thereto and wan thou haſt ycuver yt wel led yt hom and do yt in a ſoler that ſonne ne wynd may come ther'to and dimembr' it and do yt in a clene water and lef yt ther' half a day and after do yt up on herdeles for to drie and wan yt ys drye tak ſalt and do after thy veniſon axit[1] and do yt boyle in water that yt be other[m] ſo ſalt als water of the ſee and moche more and after lat the water be cold that it be thynne and thanne do thy Veniſon in the water and lat yt be therein thre daies and thre nyzt[n] and after tak yt owt of the water and ſalt it wyth drie ſalt ryzt wel in a barel and wan thy barel ys ful cuver it haſtely that ſunne ne wynd come thereto.

LVII. For to do away Reſtyn[o] of Veniſon.

Tak the Veniſon that ys reſt and do yt in cold water and after mak an hole in the herthe and lat yt be thereyn thre dayes and thre nyzt and after tak

---

[1] as thy veniſon requires. See Gloſſ to Chaucer for *axe*.
[m] Dele.
[n] A plural, as in N° 57.
[o] Reſtineſs. It ſhould be rather *reſtyng*. See below.

[ 112 ]

yt up and fpot yt wel wyth gret falt of peite [p] thete were the reftyng ys and after lat yt hange in reyn water al nyzt or mor'.

LVIII. For to make poñdorroge [q].

Tak Partrichis wit [r] longe filettis of Pork al raw and hak hem wel fmale and bray hem in a morter and wan they be wel brayed do thereto god plente of pouder and zolkys of eyryn and after mak ther'of a Farfure formed of the gretneffe of a onyoñ and after do it boyle in god breth of Buf other of Pork after lat yt kele and after do it on a broche of Hafel and do them to the fere to rofte and after mak god bature of flour' and egg' on batur' wyt and another zelow and do thereto god plente of fugur and tak a fethere or a ftyk and tak of the batur' and peynte ther'on above the applyn fo that on be wyt and that other zelow wel colourd.

### Explicit fervicium de carnibus.

[p] Pierre, or Petre.
[q] Vide N° 42.
[r] with.

*Hic incipit Servicium de Piſſibus* [a].

I. For to make Egarduſe [b].

TAK Lucys [c] or Tenchis and hak hem ſmal in gobett' and fry hem in oyle de olive and ſyth nym vineger and the thredde party of ſugur and myncyd onyons ſmal and boyle al togeder' and caſt ther'yn clowys macys and quibibz and ſerve yt forthe.

II. For to make Rapy [d].

Tak pyg' or Tenchis or other maner freſch fyſch and fry yt wyth oyle de olive and ſyth nym the cruſtys of wyt bred and canel and bray yt al wel in a mortere and temper yt up wyth god wyn and cole [e] yt thorw an herſyve and that yt be al cole [f] of canel and boyle yt and caſt ther'in hole clowys and macys

---

[a] See p. 1.

[b] See N° 21 below, and part I. N° 50.

[c] Lucy, I preſume, means the *Pike*, ſo that this fiſh was known here long before the reign of H. VIII. though it is commonly thought otherwiſe. V Gloſſ.

[d] Vide N° 49

[e] Strain, from Lat *colo*

[f] Strained, or cleared.

[ 114 ]

and quibibz and do the fyfch in difchis and rape [g]
abovyn and dreffe yt forthe.

### III. For to make Fygey.

Nym Lucys or tenchis and hak hem in morfell'
and fry hem tak vyneger and the thredde party of
fugur myncy onyons fmal and boyle al togedyr caft
ther'yn macis clowys quibibz and ferve yt forth.

### IIII. For to make Pommys morles.

Nym Rys and bray hem [h] wel and temper hem up
wyth almaunde mylk and boyle yt nym applyn and
par' hem and fher hem fmal als dicis and caft hem
ther'yn after the boylyng and caft fugur wyth al and
colowr yt wyth fafron and caft ther'to pouder and
ferve yt forthe.

### V. For to make rys moyle [i].

Nym rys and bray hem ryzt wel in a morter and
caft ther'to god Almaunde mylk and fugur and falt
boyle yt and ferve yt forth.

### VI. For to make Sowpys dorry.

Nym onyons and mynce hem fmale and fry hem in

---

[g] This Rape is what the difh takes its name from. Perhaps
means *grape* from the French *raper*. Vide N° 28

[h] Ry e, as it confifts of grains, is here confidered as a plural.
See alfo N° 5. 7, 8.

[i] Vide Gloff.

oyl dolyf Nym wyn and boyle yt wyth the onyouns tofte wyte bred and do yt in difchis and god Almande mylk alfo and do ther'above and ferve yt forthe.

VII. For to make Blomanger [k] of Fyfch.

Tak a pound of rys les hem wel and wafch and feth tyl they brefte and lat hem kele and do ther'to mylk of to pound of Almandys nym the Perche or the Lopufter and boyle yt and keft fugur and falt alfo ther'to and ferve yt forth.

VIII. For to make a Potage of Rys.

Tak Rys and les hem and wafch hem clene and feth hem tyl they brefte and than lat hem kele and feth caft ther'to Almand mylk and colour it wyth fafron and boyle it and meffe yt forth.

IX. For to make Lamprey frefch in Galentyne [l].

Schal be latyn blod atte Navel and fchald yt and roft yt and ley yt al hole up on a Plater and zyf hym forth wyth Galentyn that be mad of Galyngale gyngener and canel and dreffe yt forth.

X. For to make falt Lamprey in Galentyne [m].

Yt fchal be ftoppit [n] over nyzt in lews water and

[k] See note on N° 14 of Part I
[l] This is a made or compounded thing. See both here, and in the next Number, and v. Gloff.
[m] See note [l] on the laft Number.
[n] Perhaps, *fteppit*, i. e. fteeped. See N° 12.

in bran and flowe and fodyn and pyl onyons and feth hem and ley hem al hol by the Lomprey and zif hem forthe wyth galentyne makyth º wyth ftrong vyneger and wyth paryng of wyt bred and boyle it al togeder' and ferve yt forthe.

XI. For to make Lampreys in Bruet.

They fchulle be fchaldyd and yfode and ybrulyd upon a gredern and grynd peper and fafron and do ther'to and boyle it and do the Lomprey ther'yn and ferve yt forth.

XII. For to make a Storchon.

He fchal be fhorn in befys ᵖ and ftepyd ᵠ over nyzt and fodyn longe as Flefch and he fchal be etyn in venegar.

XIII. For to make Solys in Bruet.

They fchal be fleyn and fodyn and roftyd upon a gredern and grynd Peper and Safron and ale boyle it wel and do the fole in a plater and the bruet above ferve it forth.

XIV. For to make Oyftryn in Bruet.

They fchul be fchallyd ʳ and yfod in clene water

---

º Perhaps, *makyd*, i. e. made.
ᵖ Perhaps *pilys*, i. e. pieces
ᵠ Qu *ftepid*, i. e. fteeped.
ʳ Have fhells taken off.

grynd

grynd peper fafroñ bred and ale and temper it wyth Broth do the Oyſtryn ther'ynne and boyle it and falt it and ſerve it forth.

XV. For to make Elys in Bruet.

They fchul be flayn and ket in gobett' and fodyn and grynd peper and fafioñ other myntys and perſele and bred and ale and temper it wyth the broth and boyle it and ſerve it forth.

XVI. For to make a Lopiſter.

He fchal be roſtyd in his fcalys in a ovyn other by the Feer under a panne and etyn wyth Veneger.

XVII. For to make Porreyne.

Tak Piunys fayrift wafch hem wel and clene and frot hem wel in fyve for the Jus be wel ywronge and do it in a pot and do ther'to wyt gres and a party of fugur other hony and mak hem to boyle togeder' and mak yt thykke with flowr of rys other of waftel bred and wan it is fodyn dreffe it into difchis and ftrew ther'on powder and ferve it forth.

XVIII. For to make Chireſeye.

Tak Chiryes at the Feſt of Seynt John the Baptiſt and do away the ftonys grynd hem in a morter and after frot hem wel in a feve fo that the Jus be wel comyn owt and do than in a pot and do ther'in feyr gres

[ 118 ]

gres or Boter and bred of waſtrel ymyid [s] and of ſugur a god party and a porcion of wyn and wan it is wel yſodyn and ydreſſyd in Dyſchis ſtik ther'in clowis of Gilofr' and ſtrew ther'on ſugur.

XIX. For to make Blank de Sur' [t].

Tak the zolkys of Eggs ſodyn and temper it wyth mylk of a kow and do ther'to Comyn and Safron and flowr' of ris or waſtel bred mycd and grynd in a morter and temper it up wyth the milk and mak it boyle and do ther'to wit [u] of Egg' corvyn ſmale and tak fat cheſe and kerf ther'to wan the licour is boylyd and ſerve it forth.

XX. For to make Grave enforſe.

Tak tȳd [w] gyngener and Safron and grynd hem in a morter and temper hem up wyth Almandys and do hem to the fir' and wan it boylyth wel do ther'to zolkys of Egg' ſodyn and fat cheſe corvyn in gobettis and wan it is dreſſid in diſchis ſtrawe up on Powder of Galyngale and ſerve it forth.

XXI. For to make Hony Douſe [x].

Tak god mylk of Almandys and rys and waſch hem wel in a feyr' veſſel and in fayr' hoth water and

---

[s] Perhaps ymycd, i. e. minced, or mycd, as in N° 19.
[t] Vide Note c on N° 29. of l'art I.
[u] white. So wyt is white in N° 21. below.
[w] It appears to me to be tryd. Can it be fryd?
[x] See Part II. N° 1, and Part I. N° 50.

after

after do hem in a feyr towayl for to drie and wan that they be drye bray hem wel in a morter al to flowr' and afterward tak two partyis and do the half in a pot and that other half in another pot and colowr that on wyth the fafron and lat that other be wyt and lat yt boyle tyl it be thykke and do ther'to a god party of fugur and after dreffe yt in twe difchis and loke that thou have Almandys boylid in water and in fafron and in wyn and after frie hem and fet hem upon the fyre fethith mete [y] and ftrew ther'on fugur that yt be wel ycolouryt [z] and ferve yt forth.

XXII. For to make a Potage Feneboiles.

Tak wite benes and feth hem in water and bray the benys in a morter al to nozt and lat them fethe in almande mylk and do ther'in wyn and hony and feth [a] reyfons in wyn and do ther'to and after dreffe yt forth.

XXIII. For to make Tartys in Applis.

Tak gode Applys and gode Spycis and Figys and reyfons and Perys and wan they are wel ybrayed colourd [b] wyth Safron wel and do yt in a cofyn and do yt forth to bake wel.

[y] Seth it, mete, i. e. feeth it properly.
[z] Coloured See N° 28. below.
[a] i. e Seeth
[b] Perhaps, *coloure*.

XXIV.

[ 120 ]

XXIV. For to make Rys Alker'.

Tak Figys and Reyfons and do awey the Kernelis and a god party of Applys and do awey the paryng of the Applis and the Kernelis and bray hem wel in a morter and temper hem up with Almande mylk and menge hem wyth flowr of Rys that yt be wel chariaunt and ftrew ther'upon powder of Galyngale and ferve yt forth.

XXV. For to make Tartys of Fyfch owt of Lente.

Mak the Cowche of fat chefe and gyngener and Canel and pur' crym of mylk of a Kow and of Helys yfodyn and grynd hem wel wyth Safron and mak the chowche of Canel and of Clowys and of Rys and of gode Spycys as other Tartys fallyth to be.

XXVI. For to make Morrey[c].

Requir' de Carnibus ut fupra[d].

XXVII. For to make Flownys[e] in Lente.

Tak god Flowr and mak a Paft and tak god mylk of Almandys and flowr of is other amydon and boyle hem togeder' that they be wel chariaud wan yt is boylid thykke take yt up and ley yt on a feyr'

[c] V de Part I. N° 37.
[d] Part I N° 37.
[e] Perhaps, *Farine*, or Cuftards. Chaucer, vide *Slannis*. Fr. *Flans*.

bord

bord fo that yt be cold and wan the Cofyns ben makyd tak a party of and do upon the coffyns and kerf hem in Schiveris and do hem in god mylk of Almandys and Figys and Datys and kerf yt in fowr partyis and do yt to bake and ferve yt forth.

### XXVIII. For to make Rapee [f].

Tak the Cruftys of wyt bred and reyfons and bray hem wel in a morter and after temper hem up wyth wyn and wryng hem thorw a cloth and do ther'to Canel that yt be al colouryt of canel and do ther'to hole clowys macys and quibibz the fyfch fchal be Lucys other Tenchis fryid or other maner Fyfch fo that yt be frefch and wel yfryed and do yt in Difchis and that rape up on and ferve yt forth.

### XXIX. For to make a Porrey Chapeleyn.

Tak an hundred onyons other an half and tak oyle de Olyf and boyle togeder' in a Pot and tak Almande mylk and boyle yt and do ther'to. Tak and make a thynne Paaft of Dow and make therof as it were ryngis tak and fry hem in oyle de Olyve or in wyte grees and boil al togedere.

### XXX. For to make Formenty on a Fichfsday [g].

Tak the mylk of the Hafel Notis boyl the wete [h] wyth the aftermelk til it be dryyd and tak and colour[d][i] yt wyth Safron and the ferft mylk caft ther'to and boyle wel and ferve yt forth.

[f] Vide Part I. N° 49.  [g] Fifh.day.  [h] white.  [i] Perhaps, *colour*.

[ 122 ]

XXXI. For to make Blank de Syry [k].

Tak Almande mylk and Flowr' of Rys Tak ther'to fugur and boyle thys togeder' and difche yt and tak Almandys and wet hem in water of Sugur and drye hem in a panne and plante hem in the mete and ferve yt forth.

XXXII. For to make a Pynade or Pyvade.

Take Hony and Rotys of Radich and grynd yt fmal in a morter and do yt ther'to that hony a quantite of broun fugur and do ther'to Tak Powder of Peper and Safron and Almandys and do al togeder' boyl hem long and hord[l] yt in a wet bord and let yt kele and meffe yt and do yt forth [m].

XXXIII. For to make a Balourgly [n] Broth.

Tak Pikys and fpred hem abord and Helys zif thou haft fle hem and let hem in gobettys and feth hem in alf wyn [o] and half in water Tak up the Pykys and Elys and hold hem hote and draw the Broth thorwe a Clothe do Powder of Gyngener Peper and Galyngale and Canel into the Broth and boyle yt and do yt on the Pykys and on the Elys and ferve yt forth.

𝕰𝖝𝖕𝖑𝖎𝖈𝖎𝖙 𝖉𝖊 𝕮𝖔𝖖𝖚𝖎𝖓𝖆 𝖖𝖚𝖊 𝖊𝖘𝖙 𝖔𝖕𝖙𝖎𝖒𝖆 𝖒𝖊𝖉𝖎𝖈𝖎𝖓𝖆.

[k] V. de ad N° 29. of Part I.
[l] i. e. hap, as in next Number.
[m] This Recipe is ill expreffed
[n] This is fo uncertain in the original, that I can only guefs at it
[o] Perhaps, aif in cyr, or dele in before water.

INDEX.

# INDEX AND GLOSSARY

TO

## MR. BRANDER'S ROLL OF COOKERY.

The Numbers relate to the order of the Recipes.

N. B. Many words are now written as one, which formerly were divided, as al fo, up on, &c. Of these little notice is taken in the Index, but I mention it here once for all.

Our orthography was very fluctuating and uncertain at this time, as appears from the different modes of spelling the fame words. v. To gedre, v. wayshe, v. ynowkz, v. chargeant, v. corānte, &c.

### A.

A. abounds. a gode broth, 5. 26, al a nyzt, 192. *in.* a two, 62.
ā. and. paſſim.
Aftir. Proem. like, 176. Wiclif.
Aray. Dreſs, ſet forth, 7. Chaucer.
Alf. MS. Ed. 45. li. 33. half.
Alye it. 7. 33. mix, thicken. hence *alloy* of metals. from French *allayer*. alay, 22. aly, MS Ed. 46. See Junij Etymolog. v. Alaye. lye. here N° 15.
lyed.

[ 124 ]

lyed thickened. MS Ed. 44, 45. Randle Holme interprets lyth or lything by thickening. hence lyō. a mixture, 11. *ahth* for alyed. MS. Editor. N° 45.

Awey. MS. Ed. 27. II. 18. away.

Auance. 6 forte Avens. *Caryophylla*, Miller, Gard. Dict.

Axe. MS. Ed. N° 56. Chaucer.

Ayren. v. Eyren.

Al, Alle 23. 53. Proem. All. Chaucer. *al to breſt.* all burſt MS Ed N° 14

Als. MS. Editor. N° 29. Chaucer. in v. It means *as.*

Almandes. 17 very variouſly written at this time, Almaunde, Almandys, Almaundys, Almondes, all which occur in MS. Ed. and mean Almond or Almonds.

Almand mylke 9. Almonds blanch'd and drawn thickiſh with good broth or water, N° 51 is called *thyk mylke*, 52. and is called after Almande mylke, firſt and ſecond milk, 116. Almands unblanched, ground, and drawn with good broth, is called mylke, 62 Cow's milk was ſometimes uſed inſtead of it, as MS Ed 1 13.

Creme of Almands how made, 85. Of it, Lel. Coll. VI p. 17. We hear elſewhere of Almond-butter, v. Butter.

Azey v. 2_ ngn Lel Coll. IV. p 281. alibi. Chaucer A. S. Ægen.

Aneys, Anyſe. 36. 137 Aneys in confit rede other whyt, 36. 38. 1 e. Anis or Aniſeed confectioned red, or white uſed for garniſh, 58

Ar don. 37. v. ad locum.

Almony. 47 v. ad locum.

Almayne. 71. Germany. v. ad loc. MS. Editor, N° 2. 31.

Alkenet 47. A ſpecies of Buglos. Quincey, Diſpenſ. p. 51. 62. uſed for colouring, 51. 84. fryed and y'ondred, or yfondyt, 62. 162.

Aroon.

Anoon. 53. Anon, immediately. Wiclif.
Arn. MS. Ed. II. 23. are. Chaucer. v. *arne.*
Adoñ. 59. 85. down. v. Chaucer. voce *adoune.* MS. Edit. N° 1.
Avyfement. Proem. Advice, Direction. Chaucer. French.
Aymers. 72. Embers. Sax. æmyrian, Cineres. Belg. *ameren.*
Aquapatys. 75 a Mefs or Difh.
Alker. Rys Alker. MS. Ed. II. 24.
Appulmoy. 79. a difh. v. ad loc. Appelyn, Applys, Apples. MS. Ed. 17. 35.
Abrode. 85. abrod. MS. Ed. II. 33. abroad. So *brode.* MS. Ed. 15. broad.
Alite. v. Lite.
Ale. 113. v. Pref.
Afide. 113. apart. Wiclif.
Ayfell. 114, 115. a fpecies of Vinegar. Wiclif. Chaucer. v. *Eifel.*
Alegar. 114.
Armed. 146. v. ad loc.
Alygyn. v. Brewet.

B.

Bacon. N° 1.
Benes. 1. alibi Beans. Chaucer. v. *bene.*
Bef. 6. MS. Ed. 17. Beef. Buf, Buff. MS. Ed. 27. 42, 43.
Buth. 6. 23. 30. alibi. been, are. Chaucer has *beth.*
Ben. MS. Ed. 4. 27. be. Chaucer v. *bein* and *ben.*
Balles. 152. Balls or Pellets.
Blank Defire. 193, 194. bis. Lel. Coll. VI. p. 5. In N° 193, we meet with *Blank defire,* but the Contents has *Defire,* which is right, as appears from the fequel. In MS. Ed. 29. it is *Blank-Surry,* and *Sury,* and *Sure,* and *de Sur.* II. 19. de Syry, 31.

and here Nº 37, it is Defforre. and we have *Samon in Sorry*. Lel. Coll. VI. p. 17. Perches. ibid. Eels p. 28. 30. where it is a Potage whence I conceive it either means *de Suriey*, i. e. Syria. v. Chaucer. v. *Suriey*. Or it may mean *to be defired*, as we have *Houfys of Defyn* Lel. Coll. IV. p. 272. See Nº 63. and it is plainly written *Defire* in Godwin de Præful. p. 697. In this cafe, the others are all of them corruptions

Blank Defforre v. Blank Defire.
Blank Defne. v. Blank Defire
Berandyles MS. Ed. 27
Bred, Breed. MS. Ed. paffim. Bread
Bove. 167. Above. Chaucer. Belg. *Boven*.
Blode. 11 alibi. Blod. MS. Ed. 9 Blood.
Batō. 149. of eggs, 161 179. Batur, 28. Batour. ibid 19. Batter
Borer. MS Ed. 38. Butter.
Borage. 6.
Betes. 6. Beets. Fr. *Bete*.
Burfen. 11. name of a difh. Burfews, Nº 179, is a different difh.
Brek. MS Ed. 6. 23. break, bruſe
Breft, brefte. MS. Ed. 1. 14. burft.
Bukkennade. 17. a difh. Buknade, 118. where it means a mode of dreffing. vide MS. Ed. 45. 52.
Bryddes. 19. Briddes, 60. 62. Birds, per metathefin. Chaucer.
Brawn of Capons. 20. 84. Flefh Braun. MS. Ed. 29. v. Chaucer. we now fay, *brawn of the arm*, meaning the flefh. Hence *brawn-fall'n*. Old Plays, XI. p. 85 Lylie's Euphues, p. 94. 142 Chaucer. Brawn is now appropriated to thefe rolls which are made of Brawn or Boar, but it was not fo anciently, fince in Nº 52 we have *Brawn of Swyne*, which fhews the word was common to other kinds of

of flesh as well as that of the Boar; and therefore I cannot agree with Dr. Wallis in deducing *Brawn* from *Apiugna*.

Blank mang. 36. 192 Chaucer writes *Blank manger*. Blomanger. MS. Ed. 14 33. 34 II. 7. N B a very different thing from what we make now under that name, and see Holme, III. p. 81.

Bronchis. MS. Ed 55. Branches.

Braan. MS. Ed II. 10. Bran.

Bet MS. Ed. II. 21 Beater.

Broche. MS. Ed. 58. a Spit.

Brewet of Almony. 47. v. Almony. of Ayren, or eggs, 91. MS. Ed. 23. Eles in Brewet, 110 where it seems to be composed of Bread and Wine Muskles in Brewet, 122. Hens in Bruet, MS. Ed. 7 Cold, 131. 134 Bruet and Brewet are French *Brovet*, Pottage or Broth. Bruet riche, Lel. Coll. IV. p 226 *Beorwete*, p. 227, as I take it. *Blanche Brewet de Alyngyn*, MS. Ed. 13. 23.

Boon. 55 Bone. Chaucer.

Brenyng. 67. 188. burning, per metathesin, from *bren* or *brenne*, used by Skelton, in the Invective against Wolsey, and many old authors. Hence the disease called brenning or burning. Motte's Abridgement of Phil Transf. part IV. p 245. Reid's Abridgement, part III. p 149. Wiclif has *brenne* and *bryn* . Chaucer. v. *bren*, *Brinne*, &c.

Blake. 68 Black. Chaucer.

Berst. 70. 181. 192. burst. Chaucer. A. S. beyrtan.

Breth. 71. Air, Steam MS. Ed. N° 2. hence *brether*, breather Wiclif.

Bron. 74 brown. A. S. bpun

Butter. 81. 91. 92. 160. Boter, MS Ed. 38. and so *boutry* is Buttery. Lel. Coll. IV. p. 281. *Almonde Butter*. Lel. VI p. 6 Rabelais, IV. c. 60.

Bynethen. 92 under, beneath Chaucer. bineth.

Bolas. 95. bullace. Chaucer.

Bifore.

Bifore. 102. before. Wiclif. Matth. xiv. Chaucer has *biforne*, and byforne.

Brafey. a compound fauce, 107.

Ballac broth 109

Brymlent Tart de Brymlent. 167. v. ad loc.

Bloms. 171. Flowers, Bloffoms. Chaucer.

Bothom 173. bottom pronounced *bothom* now in the north. Chaucer. bottym, MS. Ed. 48.

Brode. 189. broad. v. abrode.

Bataiwyng 189. embatteling qu. if not mifread for *bataillyng*. See Chaucer. v. batailed.

Bord. MS. Ed II. 27. board Chaucer.

Breyt, breth. MS. Ed. 17. 58. Broth.

Blank Surry. MS Ed. 29. II 19. v. Blank Defire.

Bifmeus. MS. Ed. 16.

## C.

C. omitted. v. Cok. v. pluk. v. Pryk. v. Pekok. v Ph.fik v thyk on the contrary it often abounds, hence, fchulle, fhould, frefch, frefh, difche, difh, fchepys, fheeps; flefch, flefh, fyfch, fifh, fcher, cheer, &c. in MS Ed. v. Gl. to Chaucer v. fchal

Craftly. Proem. properly, *fecundum artem*.

Caboches. 4. alibi. Cabbages. f. Fr. Caboche, Head, Pate.

Caraway. 53. v. Junij Etymolog

Carvon. 152. carved, cut. Corvyn, MS. Ed. II 19, 20. cut. *Corve*, i. e. corve, 4. cut. v. ycorve. v. kerve.

Canell paffim Cinamon. Wiclif. v. Pref.

Cuver. MS. Ed. 56. Cover

Cumpas. v. Cumpas. i e. Compa's, 189. by meafure, or r... .. Coll IV. p. 263.

Col. 6 Cole or Colvort Belg. *kool*.

Cort. 12. name of a difh.

Culdere. MS. Ed. 25. 27. a Cullender. Span. Coladers.

Caffelys. MS. Ed. 28.

Cranes.

[ 129 ]

Cranes. 146. *Grues*. v. ad loc.
Chyballes. 12 Chibolls, 76. young Onions. Littleton. Ital *Cibolo*. Lat. Cæpula, according to Menage; and fee Lye.
Colys MS. Ed. II. fee the Pref.
Cawdel. 15. 33. Caudell, Contents. See Junius. of Muſkels or Muſcles, 124. Cawdel Ferry, 41. In E. of Devon's teaſt it is *Feny*.
Conynges. 17. Connynges, 25. Coneys, Rabbets.
Calle. 152. Cawl of a Swine.
Connat 18. a marmolade. v. ad loc.
Clowes. 20. Cloves. v. Pref.
Canuas, or Canvaſs. 178. Fr *Canevas*. Belg. *Kanefas*.
Corante Rayſons of Corante. 14. So *Raſyns of Corens*, Northumb. Book, p. 19. *Raiſin de Corinthie*. Fr. i. e. of Corinth, whence our Currants, which are ſmall Raiſins, came, and took their name. *Corance*, 17. 21. *Coraunce*, 50. *Coronſe*, MS. Ed. 42. Raiſins are called by way of contradiſtinction *grete* Rayſons, 65. 133. See Northumb. Book, p. 11.
Coronſe. v. Corante.
Chargeant. 192. Stiff. v. ad loc. MS. Fd. writes *Charchant*, 29, 30 *Charghaunt*, 33 *Charchaunt*, 34. *Chariaunt*. i. e. *Charjaunt*, 36. II. 24. *Chariand*, i. e. *Charjand*, 27.
Comyn. MS. Ed. 39.
Colure. MS. Ed. 5. to colour.
Concys. 22. ſeems to be a kind of ſauce. MS. Ed. 6. but the recipe there is different. v. ad Nº 25.
Chanke. MS. Ed. 20.
Col, Cole. 23. 52. cool. alſo to ſtrain, 70, 71. alibi. MS. Ed. II. 22. cleared.
Comyn. MS. Ed. II. 18. come.
Cowche. 24. 154. lay MS. Ed. II. 25 Chaucer, v. Couche.
Cynee. 25. a certain ſauce. perhaps the ſame with Concy. Nº 22. Plays in Cynee, 112. Sooles, 119. Tenches, 120. Oyſters, 123.

R             Harys

[ 130 ]

Harys [Hares] in Cinee. MS. Ed. 8. where doubtlefs we fhould read Cinee, fince in N° 51 there it is *Cyney*. It is much the fame as *bruet*, for *Scoles in Cynee* here is much the fame with *Solys in bruet*. MS. Ed. II. 13.

Chykens. 27. 33. Chicken is a plural itfelf. but in MS. Ed 13. it is *Chekenys* alfo, and *Chyckyns*. Lel. Coll IV. p. 1. *Checonys* MS. Ed.

Carnel of Pork. 32. v. ad loc.

Corvyn. v. Carvon.

Cu-lews. 35. not eaten now at good tables; however they occur in archb. Nevill's feaft. Lel. Coll. VI. p. 1. And fee Northumb. Book, p. 106. Rabelais iv. c. 59. And Earl of Devon's Feaft.

Confit, or Confyt. v. Aneys and Colyandre.

Charlet. 39. a difh. v. ad loc.

Chefe ruayn. 49. 166. perhaps of Rouen in Normandy. *rouen* in Fr. fignifies the colour we call *roan*.

Crems. 52. for fingular Cream. written *Creme*, 85. 183. Crem and Crym, in MS. Ed. 34. II. 24. Fr. *Crefme, Creme*

Cormarye. 53 a difh. qu.

Colyandre. 53. 128. where it is *in Confyt rede*, or red. White is alfo ufed for garnifh, 59. Celenbpe, A. S. Ciliandro, Span

Chyryfe. 58. a made difh of cherries. v. ad loc.

Cheweryes. 58. Cherries. v. ad loc. and MS. Ed. II. 18. ubi *Chiryes*.

Croton, 60. a difh. v. ad loc.

Crayton. v. Croton.

Cleeve a two. 62. cloven. A. S. cleopan.

Cyrip. 64. Sirrup. v. ad loc.

Chyches. 72. Vetches, v. ad loc.

Chawf. 74 warm. Fr. *Echauffer*, whence Chaucer has *Efchaufe*.

Clat.

Clat. 78. a diſh. qu.
Chef. Proem. chief. Fr.
Calwar Salmon. 98. v. ad loc.
Compoſt. 100. a preparation ſuppoſed to be always at hand. v. ad loc.
Comfery. 190. Comfrey. v. ad loc.
Chargeours. 101 diſhes v. ad 126.
Chyſanne. 103. to be eaten cold
Congur 104. 115. Lel Coll VI. p. 6. bis. p. 16. *Cungers* are among the fiſh in Mr. Topham's MS. for the Conger, little uſed now, ſee Pennant. III. p. 115.
Coffyns. 113. Pies raiſed without their lids, 158. 167. 185. 196. MS. Ed. II. 23. 27. In Wiclif it denotes baſkets.
Comade. 113. Comadore. 188.
Coūtour. 113 Coverture, Lid of a Pye.
Codlyng. 94. grete Codelyng, 114. v. ad loc.
Chawdōn. 115. for Swans, 143. *Swan with Chawdron*. Lel Coll. IV. p. 226. which I ſuppoſe may be true orthography. So *Swann with Chaudron*. Earl of Devon's Feaſt. And it appears from a MS. of Mr. Aſtle's, where we have among *Sawces*, *Swanne is good with Chaldron*, that *Chaldron* is a ſauce.
Crome. 131. Pulp, Kernel. Crūmes 159. Chaucer. The Crum is now the ſoft part of a loaf, oppoſed to the cruſt.
Cury. Proem. Cookery. We have aſſumed it in the title.
Camelyne. 144. a ſauce. an *Canelyne*, from the flour of Canel?
Crudds. 150. 171. Curds, per metatheſin, as common in the north
Cruſtards. 154. Pies, from the *Cruſt* quære if our *Cuſtard* be not a corruption of Cruſtard; Junius gives a different etymon, but whether a better, the Reader muſt judge. Cruſtard of fiſh, 156. of herbs, 157.

157 and in the Earl of Devon's Feast we have *un Pyte Cryspade*.

Cryspes. 162. Cryspels. 163. v. ad loc *Fritter Crispayne*. Ll. Coll VI. p 5. which in Godwin de Praeful p 697. is *Frater Crispin*

Chawfō. 162. Cowfer, 173. a Chafing-dish. Chafer. Lel Coll IV. p. 302 v. Junius voce *Chafe*.

Curose. 171. curiously perhaps from *cure*, to cook. Chaucer has *corouse*, curious.

Clarry. 172. Clary.

Coragres. 175. a dish. v ad loc.

Cok. 75. a Cock. &c, Lel. Coll. IV. p 227.

Chewets. 185. 186 a dish Rand Holme, III. p. 78. 81, 82. Birch, Life of Prince Henry, p. 458.

Comadore v. Comade.

Chastlet. 189. v. ad loc.

Christen Proem. Christian.

### D.

Do. 1, 2 put, cause MS Ed. 2. 12. Chaucer. *make*. 56. done, 48. So Chaucer has *do* for *done*.

Dof. do off. 101.

Draw. drawen 2. strained. hence 3. 20. 23. *drawe the grewel thurgh a straynour*.
 To boil. 2. 17. as, *drawe hem up with gode brothe*. also 51. 74.
 To put, 14. 41.
 To make. 28 47. as, *draw an Almande mylke*.

Dee. 152. singular of Dice, the Fr. Dè. v. quare.

Drepe. 19 a dish. qu.

Dates. 20. 52 158. the fruit.

Dish. 2. dish.

Desforre. 37. v. Blank desire.

Doust. 45. alibi Dust.

Dowhz,

Dowhz. 50. Dowh. 92. Dow. MS. Ed. II. 29. Dough, Paste. A. S *bah*.
Douce Ame. 63. quasi a delicious dish. v. Blank Desire.
Drope. 67. drop. to baste. MS. Ed 28.
Dorry. Sowpes dorry, 82. Sops endorsed. from *endore*, 187. MS. Ed. 42. II. 6. vide ad 174.
Deel 113 170. part, some. v. Sum. Chaucer.
Dicayn. 172. v. ad loc
Dokks. as *Sowre Dokks*, 173 Docks.
Dorryle. v. Pome.
Daryols. 183. a dish. A Custard baked in a Crust. Hear Junius, v Dairie. 'G. *dariole* dicitur hbi 'genus, quod iisdem Gallis alias nuncupatur *laic-* '*teron* vel *flan de laict.*'
Desne. v Blank Desire.
Desire. v. Blank.
Dressit. 194. dressed. dresse. MS. Ed. 15. et passim. Chaucer in voce. hence ydressy. MS. Ed. II. 18.
Dysis MS. Ed. 15 dice. v quare
Demembre, dimembre. MS. Ed. 31. dismember.
Dows, douze. MS. Ed 50. II. 21.
Drong. MS. Ed. 54. drunk.

E.

E. with *e* final after the consonant, for *ea*, as brede, bread; benes, beans, bete, beat, breke, break, creme, cream, clere, clear, clene, clean; mede, mead; mete, meat, stede, stead, whete, wheat; &c

E with *e* final after the consonant, for *ee*, as betes, beets; chese, cheese, depe, deep, fete, feet; grene, green; nede, needful, swete, sweet.
Endorre. MS. Ed 42 endorse.
Ete. 10&. eat *eten*, 146. eaten. *etyn*. MS. Ed. 3. A. S. etan. MS. Ed. 48. eat.

Ensorse.

Enforse. MS. Ed. II. 20 seasoned.
Erbes. 7 herbs, *herbes*, 63. *erbys*, 151. Eerbis, 157.
Eyren, and Ayren. 7, 8 15 Eyryn, MS Ed. 1 Eggs.
 ‘ a merchant at the N Foreland in Kent asked for
 ‘ eggs, and the good wyf answerede, that she coude
 ‘ speak no Frenshe — another sayd, that he wolde
 ‘ have *eyren*, then the good wyf sayd that she un-
 ‘ derstood hym wel.’ Caxton's Virgil, in Lewis'
 Life of Caxton, p. 61. who notes ‘ See Sewel's
 ‘ Dictionary, v. *Ey*.’ add, Urry's Chaucer. v. Aye
 and Eye Note here the old plural *en*, that *eggs* is
 sometimes used in our Roll, and that in Wiclif *eye*,
 or *e*, is the singular, and in the *Germ*. See Chaucer.
 v *Are*, and *Ay*.
Eowts. 6. v. ad loc.
Egurdouce. 21. v. ad loc. of Fysshe, 133. Egge dows,
 MS Ed 50. male. Egerdufe. ibid. II. 1 Our N°
 58, is really an Lagerdouce, but different from this
 here A Seville Orange is Aigre-douce. Cotgrave.
Esy 67. easy. eselich, 113 easily. Chaucer.
Eny. 74 173 any.
Elena Campana. 78 i. e. Enula Campana, *Elecampane*.
Erbowle 95. a dish v. ad loc.
Erbolat. 172 a dish. v ad loc.
Lerys, Eris. 177. 182. 55. Ears. *Eyr*. MS. Ed. 44.
 Chaucer has *Ere* and *Eris*.
Elren. 171. Elder. *Eller*, in the north, without *d*.
Erne. 174 qu.
Euarund. MS. Ed. 3.
Eelys. 101. Eels. *Lys*, *Helys*. MS. Ed. II. 15. 24.
 *Elis* Chaucer.

F.

Forced. 3. farced, stuft. we now say, *forc'd meat*,
 yfarced, 159, 160. *enforsed*. MS. Ed. II. 20. *fors*,
 170.

[ 135 ]

170. called *fars*, 150. it seems to mean *season*, N° 4.

    Mixt. 4. where potage is said to be *forced* with powdō-douce.

Fort. passim. strong. Chaucer.

Fresee. MS. Ed. 47.

Fenkel. 6. 77. *Fenel*, 76 172. *Fenell*, 100. Fennel. Germ. Venikol. Belg. Venckel.

Fome Proem 95. forme.

Funges. 10. Mushrooms, from the French Cotgrave. Holme III. p. 82. The Romans were fond of them.

Fesants 20. 35

Fynelich wel. 192. very wel, constantly.

Fro. 22. MS. Ed. 55. Chaucer. from. So therfro. 53. Lel. Coll. IV. p. 266. Chaucer.

Fleysch. 24. Fleissh, 37. Flesh, A. S. flæysc. Germ. *Fleisc*.

Feneboyles. MS. Ed. II. 22.

Fyletts 28. Fillets.

Florish and Flō. 36. 38. 40. Garnish. Lel. Coll. VI. p 17. 23. Chauc r. v. Floure.

Foyles. 49. rolled Paste. *Foyle of dowhz*, 50. 92. et per se, 148. 153 *Foile of Paste*, 163. Leaves of Sage, 161. Chaucer. v. ad 175. hence Carpe in Foile. Lel. Coll. IV. p. 226. *a Dolphin in Foyle, a suttletie*. VI. p. 5. *Lyng in Foyle*, p. 16. *Cunger*. Ibid. *Samon*. Ibid. *Sturgen*. p. 17. et v. p. 22. N. B. Foyle in these cases means Paste.

Fars. v. forced.

Fle 53. flea, flaw. MS. Ed. II. 33. flawe, fleir, flain, flawed. 10. 13. 15.

Fonnell 62 a dish.

Frot. MS. Ed. II. 17. rub, shake, *frote*, Chaucer.

Feyre. 66 MS. Ed. II. 18. 22. *Feir*. Chaucer. Fair.

Ferthe. 68. Fourth. hence Ferthing or Farthing.

Furmente. 69. 116. *Furmenty*. MS. Ed. 1. *Formetc*. Ibid. 48. *Formenty*, Ib. II. 30. from Lat. *Frumentum*,

[ 136 ]

*tum*, per metathesin; whence called more plausibly *Frumity* in the north, and Frumetye in Lel Collect. IV. p. 226. VI. p. 5. 17. 22. but see Junius, v. Formetie.

Frenche. 73. a dish. v. ad loc.

Fest. MS. II. 18. Feast. Chaucer.

Fygey. 89. because made of Figs. Fygs drawen. 103. MS. Ed II. 3.

Found. 93 mix. dissolve, 193. fond. 188. v. y fonded. Lye, in Junii Etym. v. Founder.

Fete. 102. Chaucer. Fet, MS. Ed. 44. Feet.

Flaumpeyns. 113 184.

Ferst. MS. Ed. II 30. First.

Fanne. 116. to fan or winnow. A. S. fann, Vannus.

Frytō. 149, 150, 151. Fruturs. MS. Ed. 19 40. Fritters. *Fruter*, Lel. Coll. IV. p. 227. Frytor. VI. p. 17.

Flaunne. 163. Flownys. MS. Ed. II. 27. Fr. Flans, Custards. Chaucer. v. Slaunnis. Et v. Junium voce *Flawn*.

Feel. 168. hold, contain. perhaps same as *feal*, occultare, abscondere, for which see Junii Etymol

Fuyr. 188. Fire. *Fyr fort*. 192. a strong Fire. *Fere*, Chaucer. *Fyer*, Lel. Coll. IV. p. 296. Belg. *Vuyr*. *Fere*. MS. Ed. 58.

Ferry. v. Cawdel.

Flowr, Flowre. MS. Ed. 2. 19. Flour.

Fronchemoyle. MS Ed. 15.

Froys. MS. Ed. 18. Fraise.

Farsure. MS Ed. 28. stuffing.

Forsy. MS. Ed. 38. season.

### G.

Gronden 1. 53. ground or beaten. *to grynde* is to cut or beat small. 3. 8. 13. for compare 14. ygrōnd 37. 53. 105. to pound or beat in a mortar. 3. MS. Ed. 5.

Gode.

[ 137 ]

Gode. N° 1. alibi. good, strong. Chaucer. *god*, MS. Ed. passim.

Grete. mynced. 2. not too small. *gretust*, 189. greatest. *gret*, MS. Ed. 15. and Chaucer.

Gourdes. 8. Fr. gouhourde.

Gobettes. 16. 62. Gobbettys, Gobettis. MS. Ed. 9. alibi. Chaucer. *Gobbins*, Holme III. p. 81, 82. large pieces. Wiclif. Junii Etym.

Grees. 17. 101. Grece, 18. alibi. MS Ed. 8. 14. 32. alibi. whyte Grece, 18. Fat, Lard, Conys of high Grece. Lel. Coll. IV. p. 226. qu.

Gravey. 26, 27. *Grave.* MS. Ed. II. 20. *Gravy.* Lel. Coll. VI. p. 10.

Galyntyne. 28. 117. a preparation seemingly made of Galingale, &c. 129. and thence to take its name. See a recipe for making it, 138. as also in MS. Ed. 9. Bread of Galyntyne, 94. Soupes of Galyntyne, 129. Lampervey in Galantine. Lel. Coll. IV. p. 226. VI. p. 22. Swanne, VI. p. 5.

Garlete and Garlec. 30. 34. Garlick. A. S. ȝarleac.

Grapes. 30. 34.

Galyngale. 30. the Powder, 47 the long-rooted Cyperus. Gl. to Chaucer. See Northumberland Book, p. 415.

Gleyr̄. of Ayrĕn. 59. the white, from Fr. glaire. Chaucer. *Lear* or *Leir* of an Egg. Holme interprets it *the White beaten into a foam.*

Goon. 59. MS. Ed. 1. go. Belg. *goen.*

Gylofre. 65. Gelofre. MS. Ed. 27. cloves; for see N° 30, 31. 40. there, from Gr. καρυόφυλλον.

Gyngawdry 94. a dish.

Grave. MS. Ed. II. 20. Gravey.

Gele. 101, 102. Jelly. Fr. Gelee

Gawdy Grene. 112. perhaps, Light Green.

Gurnards. 115.

Greynes de Parys. 137. and so Chaucer, meaning *Greynes de paradys*, or greater Cardamoms. See Dr.

S            **Percy**

[ 138 ]

Percy on Northumb. Book, p. 414. Chaucer has *Greines* for *Grains*, and Belg. Greyn.

Grate. 152 v. i or y grated.

Gaftbon. 194. f. *Gaftbon*, quafi *Waftbon*, from *Waftel* the fineft Bread, which fee. Hence the Fr. Gafteau.

Gyngynyr, Gyngenyr, Gyngyner, Gyngener. MS. Ed. 3, 4. 13. 24. Ginger. Gyngyner-bred, 32.

Grotys. MS. Ed. II. Oat-meal Grotes, i. e. Grits.

Grydern, Gryder, Gredern. MS. Ed. 25 44. II. 11.

### H.

H. for *th*, as hem, them, her, their, paffim. *Hare*, 121. Chaucer. Wiclif. It is fometimes omitted; as *wyt* and *wyte*, white. Sometimes abounds, as fchaldyd. MS Ed. 7 11. fcalded. v. *Thowehe*.

Hye. Proem. high. *hy*, MS Ed. 44. A. S. Heah.

Hē. 1, 2 i e. hem; them. Lye in Junii Etym.

Hulle. 1. a verb, to take off the hufk or fkin. Littleton Hence Hulkes, Hufks or *Hulls*, as 71. *Holys*, MS. Ed. 1. Sax. helan, to cover. v. Lye in Junii Etym. v. Hull.

Hulkes. v Hulle.

Hewe. 7. cut, mince. *yheue*, 12. minced. hewn. MS. Ed. 6. 9. *hewin*, Chaucer. A. S. hepyan.

Hakke. 194. MS. Ed. 23. hack, bruife. Junii Etym. v. hack. MS. Ed. has alfo *hak* and *hac*.

Hebolace. 7. name of a difh.

Herdeles MS. Ed. 56 Hurdles.

Hennes. 17. 45 including, I prefume, the whole fpecies, as *Malard* and *Polok* do below.

Hool. 20. 22. alibi. *hole*, 33. 175 *hoole*, 158. whole. Chaucer has hole, hool, and hoolich; and Wiclif, *hole* and *hool*. MS. Ed. has *hol* and *hole*.

Hooles. 162. Holes.

Holfomly.

[ 139 ]

Holsomly. Proem. wholesomely.
Herthe. MS. Ed. 57. Earth.
Hit. 20. 98. 152. it. hytt. Northumb. Book, p. 440. *Hit*, Gloss. Wiclif. in Marg. A. S. hiτ.
Hoot. 21. alibi. hot.
Hares. 23.
Hoggepot. 31. v. ad loc.
Hochee. 34. hachè, Fr. but there is nothing to intimate cutting them to pieces.
Herfyve. MS. Ed. II. 2. Hair-sieve. *her* is *hair* in Chaucer.
Helde. 50. 154. throw, cast, put. v. 189. *Heelde*, poured, shed. Wiclif. and Lye in Junii Etym. v. Held.
Holde. 189. make, keep. MS. Ed. II. 32, 33.
Hawtheen. 57. Hawthorn. Junius, v. Haw.
Hatte. 59. bubling, wallop. quasi *the hot*, as in Chaucer. from A. Sax. haττ.
Hong. 67. hing, or hang. Chaucer. MS. Ed. 48.
Honde. 76. hand. Chaucer. So in Derbyshire now.
Heps. 84. Fruit of the Canker-rose. So now in Derbyshire, and v. Junius, voce *Hippes*.
Hake. 94. 186. a Fish. v. ad loc.
Hilde. 109. to skin, from to hull. to scale a fish, 119. vide 117. 119. compared with MS. Ed. II. 13.
Herons. 146. MS. Ed. 3. Holme, III. p. 77, 78. but little used now. Heronsew. Lel. Coll. IV. p. 226. *Heronshawe.* VI p. 1. Heronsews. Chaucer The Poulterer was to have in his shop *Ah deas five airones*, according to Mr. Topham's MS. written about 1250. And *Heronns* appear at E. of Devon's Feast.
Holke. 173. qu hollow.
Hertrowee. 176. a dish. *Hert* is *the Hart* in Chaucer. A. S. heoητ.
Hi. MS. Ed. 27. they.
Hevyd. MS Ed. 21. v. ad loc.
Hom. MS. Ed. 56. Home.

I.

## I.

I. 2. for e. Proem. So *ith* for *eth*. Ibid.
I. 30. et sæpius. in. *inne*, 37. alibi.
Jushell. 43. a dish. v. ad loc.
Is. plur. for es. 52. 73. Proem. Nomblys. MS. Ed.
  12. Nombles. v. Pees. Rosys, 177, Roses.
I. for y. v. y.
Iowtes. v. Eowtes.
Irne. 107. *Iren*, Chaucer. and the Saxon. Iron.
Juys. 118. 131. *Jus*, MS. Ed. II. 17. the Fr. word,
  *Ieuse*, Chaucer.

## K.

Kerve. 8. cut. *kerf*, 65 MS Ed. 29. v. carvon, and
  Chaucer. voc. Carfe, karft, kerve, kerft.
Kydde. 21. Flesh of a Kid. Kedys. MS. Ed. 13. Kids.
Keel. 29. 167. 188. MS. Ed. 1. Gl. to Chaucer and
  Wiclif, to cool.
Kyt. 118. alibi. MS. Ed. 19. *ket*, Ibid II. 15. to cut.
  *kyted*, cut. Lel. Coll IV. p. 298. Chaucer. v. *Kitt*.
Keintlick. v. queintlick.
Kyrnels 189. a species of battlements, from *kernellare*;
  for which see Spelman, Du Fresne, and Chaucer.
Kever. MS. Ed. 2. cover.
Kaste, kest. MS. Ed. 6. 10. cast. v. ad loc.
Kow. MS. Ed. 38. Cow.

## L.

L. for ll. MS. Ed. sæpe.
Lat. 9. 14. alibi. MS Ed. 1, 2. Let. Chaucer. Belg.
  *laten. latyn*. MS. Ed. II. 9. *let*.

Lire,

[ 141 ]

Lire, and Lyre. 3. 14. 45. MS. Ed. fæpe. the fleſhy part of Meat. A. S. lipe. See Lyre in Junii Etymol. Alſo a mixture, as *Dough of Bread and raw Eggs*, 15. hence ' drawe a Lyre of Brede, ' Blode, Vyneg, and Broth,' 25. So Lyō and Layō. 11. 31. all from *lye*, which ſee. Lay ſeems to mean *mix*, 31. as *layour* is mixture, 94.

Lye it up. 15. to mix; as *alye*, which ſee.

Leke. in ſing. 10. 76. Leeks.

Langdebef. 6. an herb. v. ad loc. *Longdobeef* Northumberland Book. p. 384. Bugloſs.

Lytel. 19. paſſim. *Litul* and *litull*, 104. 152. ' a litel ' of Vynegar,' 118. of Lard, 152.

Loſeyns, Loſyns. 24. 92. on fiſh-day, 128. a Lozenge is interpreted by Cotgrave, ' a little ſquare Cake of preſerved herbs, flowers, &c.' but that ſeems to have no concern here. *Lozengs* Lel. Coll. IV. p. 227.

Lyche. 152. like. *licht*. Wiclif. *lich*. Chaucer. *ylich*. Idem.

Lombe. 62. Lamb. hence Wiclif, *Lomberen*, Lambs. Chaucer, and Germ.

Leche Lumbard. 65. from the country doubtleſs, as the muſtard, N° 100. See alſo Lel. Coll. VI. p. 6. 26. *Leches*. MS. Ed. 15. are Cakes, or pieces. Rand Holme makes *Leach*, p. 83. to be ' a kind ' of Jelly made of Cream, Iſing-glaſs, Sugar, and ' Almonds, &c.' The *Leſſches* are fried, 158. v. y¹eeſhyd. *Leyſe Damaſk*. Lel. Coll. IV. p. 226. *Leche baked*. VI. p. 5. Partriche Leiche. Ibid. *Leche Damaſke*. Ibid. See alſo, p. 10. *Leche Florentine*, p. 17 *Leche Comfort*. Ibid. *Leche Gramor*. Ibid. Leche Cypres, p. 26. which in Godwin de Præful. p. 697. is *Sipers*, malè.

Lete Lardes. 68. v. ad loc.

Lave. 76. waſh.

Leyne. 82. a Layer.

Lewe

Lewe water. 98. Lews water, MS. Ed. II. 10. warm; see Gloss. to Wiclif. and Junius. v. Lukewarm.

Lumbard Muftard. 100. from the country. v. Leche. how made, N° 145

Lef. MS. Ed. 56. leave. *Lefe*, Chaucer.

Lite. 104. a few, *alite*, as they fpeak in the North. Chaucer, v. Lite, and Lyte, and Mr. Lye in his Junius.

Laumpreys. 126. Lampreys an Eel-like Sea Fifh. Pennant, Brit. Zool. III. p. 68.

Laumprons. 127 the *Pride*. Pennant, Ibid. p. 61. See Lel. Coll. VI. p. 6. 17. bis 23. Mr. Topham's MS. has *Murenulas five Lampridulas*.

Looches, Loches. 130. 133. the fifh.

Lardes of Swyne. 146. i. e. of Bacon. hence *lardid*, 147. and *Lardons*. MS. Ed. 3. 43. from the Fr. which Cotgrave explains *Slices of Lard*, i. e. Bacon, vide ad 68.

Lorer tr. MS. Ed. 55. Laurel tree. Chaucer.

Lyuōs. 152. Livers. A. S. lyrep.

Led. MS. Ed. 56. carry. *lide*, Chaucer.

Lenton. 158. Lent.

Lyng. 159. longer. Chaucer has *lenger* and *lengir*. v. Lange.

Lopufter, Lopifter. MS. Ed. II. 7. 16. v. Junii Etymolog.

Luft. as, hym luft Proem. he likes. Chaucer. v. Left.

Lewys. MS. Ed. 41. Leaves. Lefe, Chaucer. v. Lef.

Lie Liquor. Chaucer. MS. Ed 48.

Ley. MS. Ed. 6. lay.

Lefe, les. MS. Ed. 14. II. 7, 8. pick. To *leafe*, in Kent, is to glean.

## M.

Make. 7 MS. Ed. 12. 43. II. 12. to drefs. *make forth*, 102. to do. MS. Ed. II. 35.

Monchelet.

Monchelet. 16. a dish.
Mylk, Melk. MS. II. 30. Milk of Almonds, 1. 10. 13. alibi.
Moton. 16. MS. Ed. 1. Mutton. See Lel. Coll. IV. p. 226. Flemish. *Motoen.*
Mawmenee. 20. 193. a dish. v. ad loc. how made, 194. *Mamane.* Lel. Coll. IV. p. 227. Mamonie. VI. p. 17. 22. royal, 29. Manmene. MS. Ed. 29, 30. *Mamenge.* E. of Devon's Feast.
Morterelys. v. Mortrews.
Medle. 20 50 alibi. to mix. Wiclif. Chaucer.
Messe. to messe the dyshes, 22. messe forth, 24.
Moire. 38. MS. Ed. 37. ll. 26. a dish. v. ad loc.
Mortrews. 45. *Mortrews blank*, 46. of fish, 125. *Morterelys*, MS. Ed. 5. where the recipe is much the same. ' meat made of boiled hens, crummed bread, ' yolk of eggs, and safron, all boiled together,' Speght ad Chaucer. So called, says Skinner, who writes it *mortress*, because the ingredients are all pounded together in a mortar.
Moscels. 47. Morsels. Chaucer has *Morcills*. Moscels is not amiss, as *Mossil* in Chaucer is the muzle or mouth.
Mete. 67. A S. and Chaucer. Meat *Meetis*, Proem. Meats. It means also *properly*, MS. Ed. II. 21. Chaucer.
Myng. 68. MS. Ed. 30. *ming*, 76. *meng*, 127. 158. MS. Ed. 32. Chaucer. to mix. So *mung*, 192. is to stir. Wiclif. v Mengyng. A. S. menʒan.
Morow at Morow. 72. in the Morring MS. Ed. 33 a Morrow, Chaucer. on the Morow. Lel. Coll. IV. p. 234.
Makke. 74. a dish.
Meel, Mele. 86. 97. Meal. *Melis*, Meals. Chaucer. Belg. *Meel.*
Macrows. 62. Maccharone. vide ad locum.
Makerel. 106.

Muskles,

Muſkles, Muſkels. 122. Muſcles. A. S. *muſcule.*

Malard, Maulard. 141. meaning, I preſume, both ſexes, as ducks are not otherwiſe noticed. Holme, III. p. 77. and Mr. Topham's MS.

Mylates, whyte. 153. a diſh of pork, 155.

Myddell. 170. midle. *myddes.* 175. the ſame.

Mawe. 176. Stomach of a Swine. Chaucer. Junii Etym.

Moold 177. Mould.

Maziozame. 191. Marjoram. See the various orthographies in Junius, v. Majoram.

Male Marrow. 195. qu.

Moyle. v. Ris. v. Fronchemoyle.

Mulberries. 99. 132. v. Morree.

Myce, myſe. MS. Ed. 8 15. mince. myed. II. 19. minced. ymyed, 35. for ymyced. myney, II. 3. myneyd, II. 1

Mo. MS. Ed. 38. more. Chaucer.

Maner. *of* omitted. MS. Ed. 45. 47, 48. II. 2. 28.

Mad, ymad. MS. Ed. II. 9. made.

Mychil MS. Ed. 48 much. Chaucer. v. moche. Junius v. mickel.

Myntys. MS. Ed. II. 15. Mint. *Myntys,* Brit.

## N.

A Noſt 1. craſis of *an Oſte,* or Kiln; frequent in Kent, where *Hop-oſte* is the kiln for drying hops. ' Ooſt or Eaſt: the ſame that kiln or kill, Somer-
' ſetſhire, and elſewhere in the weſt,' Ray. So *Brytboſt* is a Brick-kiln in Old Pariſh-Book of *Wye* in Kent, 34 H. VIII. ' We call *eſt* or *oſt* the place in
' the houſe, where the ſmoke ariſeth, and in ſome
' manors *auſtrum* or *oſtrum* is that, where a fixed
' chimney or flew anciently hath been,' Ley, in Hearne's Cur. Diſc. p. 27 *Manors* here means, I
ſuppoſe,

Suppose manor houses, as is common in the north. Hence *Haifter*, for which see Northumb. Book, p. 415. 417. and Chaucer. v. Eftris.

Noumbles. 11. 13. Entrails of any beast, but confined now to those of a deer. I suspect a crasis in the case, quasi *an Umble*, singular for what is plural now, from Lat. *Umbilicus*. We at this day both say and write *Umbles*. Nombles, MS. Ed. 12. where it is *Nomblys of the venyson*, as if there were other Nomblys beside. The Fr. write Nombles.

Non. 68. no. Chaucer. A. S. nan.

Nyme. 114. take, *recipe*. Sax. niman. Chaucer. used in MS. Ed. throughout. See Junius. v. Nim

Notys. 144. Wallenotes, 157. So *Not*, MS. Ed. II. 30. Chaucer. Belg. *Note*.

Nyfebek. 173. a dish. quasi, nice for the *Bec*, or Mouth.

Nazt, nozt. MS. Ed. 37. not.

## O.

Oynons. 2. 4. 7. Fr. Oignons. Onions.

Orage. 6. Orache.

Other, oother. 13, 14. 54. 63. MS Ed. sæpe. Chaucer. Wiclif. A. S. oþer. or.

On, oon. 14. 20. alibi. in. as in the Saxon. *One* MS. Ed. 58. II. 21. Chaucer.

Obleys. 24. a kind of Wafer. v. ad loc.

Onys. MS. Ed. 37. once. *ones*, Chaucer. v. *Atones*, and *ones*.

Onoward, onaward. 24. 29. 107. onward, upon it.

Of. omitted, as powder Gynger, powder Gylofre, powder Galyngale. abounds, v. Lytel.

Oot. 26. alibi. Oat. Otyn. MS. Ed. II. Oaten.

Opyn. MS. Ed. 28. open.

Offall. 143. *Exta*, Giblets.

Oyftryn.

Oyſtryn. MS. Ed. II. 14. Oyſters.
Of. Proem. bv.
Ochepot. v. Hochepot.
Ovene. 1. Oven. A. S. oꝼen. Belg. Oven. *Ovyn*, MS. Ed. II. 16.
Olyve, de Olvve, Olyf, Dolyf, MS. Ed. Olive.
Owyn. MS. Ed. 22. own.

### P.

Plurals increaſe a ſyllable, Almandys, Yolkys, Cranys, Pecokys, &c. So now in Kent in words ending in *ſt*. This is Saxon, and ſo Chaucer.
Plurals in *n*, Piſyn, Hennyn, Appelyn, Oyſtrin.
Powdō douce 4. Pref.
Powdō fort. 10, 11. v. Pref.
Paſturnakes. 5. ſeems to mean *Parſnips* or Carrots, from *Paſtinaca*. *Paſternak of Rajens*. 100. of Apples, 149. means Paſtes, or Paties.
Perſel 6. 29. alibi *Perſele* MS. Ed. II. 15. Fr. *Perſil*. Parſley. Parcyle. MS. Ed. 32.
Pyke, pike. 18, 76. pick Chaucer. v. Pik.
Pluk. 76. pluck, pull. A. S. pluccian.
Pellydore. 19. v. ad loc.
Peletour 104. v. ad 19.
Paaſt. MS. Ed. II. 29. Paſte.
Potell. 20. Pottle
Pynes 20. alibi. v. Pref.
Pecys. 21. alibi. *Pece*, 190. *Pecis*, MS. Ed. 12. Chaucer. Pieces, Piece. 1.
Pep. 21 152. MS. Ed 16. has *Pepyr*. Pip 140 143. MS. Ed. 9. *Pepper*. A. S peopoꝛ and pipoꝛ.
Pap..e 24. a kind of ſauce. probably from *Papp*, a kind of P..ada
P.. Piſyn. MS. Ed. 2. Peaſe.

Peers.

[ 147 ]

Peers. 130. 138. *Pers*, 167. Perys, MS. Ed. II. 23. Pears. Pery, a Pear tree, Chaucer.

Poffynet. 30. 160. a Pofnet.

Partruches. 35. 147 *Partyches*, Contents. Partridges. *Perteryche* E. of Devon's Feaft.

Panne. 39. 50. a Pan. A.S. Panna.

Payndemayn. 60. 139. where it is *pared*. Flour. 41. 162. 49. white Bread. Chaucer.

Par. MS. Ed. 19. pare.

Peions. 18. 154. Pigeons. If you take *i* for *j*, it anfwers to modern pronunciation, and in E. of Devon's Feaft it is written *Pejonns*, and *Pyjonns*

Pynnonade. 51. from the Pynes of which it is made. v. Pynes *Pynade* or *Pivade*. MS. Ed. II. 32.

Pryk. 53 prick.

Peftels. 56 Legs We now fay *the Peftels of a lark.* of ven'fon, Lel. Collect. IV. p. 5. Qu. a corruption of *Pedeftals*.

Payn foindew. 59 *fondew*, Contents. v. ad loc.

Pefkodde. 65. Hull or Pod of Peafe, ufed ftill in the North. v Coddis in Wiclif, and Coddes in Junii Etymolog

Payn Ragōn. 67. a difh. qu.

Payn puff, or puf. 196. *Payne puffe*. E. of Devon's Feaft.

Pownas. 68. a colour. qu. v. Preface.

Porpays, Porpeys. 69. 108. falted, 116. roafted, 78. *Porpus* or Porpoife. *Porpecia*, Spelm. Gl. v. Geafpecia, which he corrects *Seafpecia*. It is furprifing he did not fee it muft be *Grafpecia* or *Crafpifcis*, i. e. *Gros* or *Craffus Pifcis*, any large fifh, a common term in charters, which allow to religious houfes or others the produce of the fea on their coafts See Du Cange in vocibus. We do not ufe the Porpoife now, but both thefe and Seals occur in Archb Nevill's Feaft. See Rabelais, IV. c. 60. and I conceive that the *Balænæ* in Mr. Topham's MS. means the Porpus.

Purey. 70. v. ad loc.

T 2

Peſon. 70, 71. *Pyſe, Pyſyn.* MS. Ed. 2. Peaſe. Brit. *Pyſen.*

Partye. 71. *a partye,* i. e. ſome. MS. Ed. 2. Chaucer.

Porrectes. 76. an herb. v. ad loc.

Purſlarye. 75. Purſlain.

Pochee. 90. a diſh of poached Eggs. v. Junius, voce *Poach.*

Powche. 94 Crop or Stomach of a fiſh. *Paunches,* 114, 115.

Pyke. 101. the fiſh. v. ad loc.

Plavs. 101 103. 112. Plaiſe; the fiſh. *Places,* Lel. Coll VI. p 6.

Pelettes. 112. Balls, Pellets. Pelotys. MS. Ed. 16.

Paunch. v. Powche.

Penne. 116 a Feather, or Pin. MS. Ed. 28. Wiclif. v. Pennes.

Pekok. 147. Peacock. *Pekokys,* MS. Ed. 4. where ſame direction occurs. Pekok. Lel. Coll. IV. p. 227.

p̄ſſe. 150. to preſs. Chaucer.

Pyner. 155. qu. v. Pref.

Prunes. 164. Junius in v. *Prunes and Damyſyns.* 167. *Prunes Damyſyns.* 156. 158. *Primes,* 169. ſhould be corrected *Prunes.* Prunys, MS. Ed. II. 17. *Prognes.* Lel. Coll. VI. p. 17. *Prune Orendge,* an Orange Plumb, p. 23. *Prones,* Northumb. Book, p. 19. plant it with Prunes, 167. ſtick it, Lel. Coll VI. p. 5. 16 22. As the trade with Damaſcus is mentioned in the Preface, we need not wonder at finding the Plumbs here.

Primes v. Prunes.

Prews of gode paſt. 176. qu.

Potews. 177. a diſh named from the pots uſed.

Pety puant. 195. *Petypanel, a marchpayne.* Lel. Coll. VI p 6.

Parade hole parade. 195. qu.

Plater. MS. Ed. II. 9. Platter.

Puff. v. Payn.

Phiſik. Proem. Phyſick.

Pomo

[ 149 ]

Pomegarnet. 84. Poungarnetts, MS. Ed. 39. Powmis gernatys. Ibid. 27. Pomgranates, per metathesin.
Penche. MS. Ed. 36.
Partyns. MS. Ed. 38. Parts.
Pommedorry. MS. Ed. 42. Poundorroge, 58. *Pomes endoryd.* E. of Devon's Feast.
Pommys morles. MS. Ed. II. 3.
Porreyne. MS. Ed. II. 17. Porrey Chapeleyn, 29.

## Q.

Quare. 5. It seems to mean to quarter, or to square, to cut to pieces however, and may be the same as to *dyce.* 10. 60. Dice at this time were very small: a large parcel of them were found under the floor of the hall of one of the Temples, about 1764, and were so minute as to have dropt at times through the chinks or joints of the boards. There were near 100 pair of ivory, scarce more than two thirds as large as our modern ones. The hall was built in the reign of Elizabeth. To *quare* is from the Fr. quarrer, and *quayre* or *quaire*, subst. in Chaucer, Skelton, p. 91. 103. is a book or pamphlet, from the paper being in the quarto form. See Annal. Dunstap p. 215 Ames, Typ. Antiq. p 39. Hence our quire of paper. The later French wrote *cahier, cayer,* for I presume this may be the same word. Hence, *kerve hem to dyce,* into small squares, 12. *Dysis,* MS Ed 15.
Quybibes. 64 Quibinz. MS. Ed 54. alibi. Cubebs.
Quenthen. 162. keyntlich, 189. nicely, curiously. Chaucer. v. *Queinthe.*
Quayle. 162. perhaps, cool. it seems to mean fail or miscarry. Lel. oll. VI. p 11. sink or be dejected, p. 41. See Junius, v. Quail.
Queynchehe. 173. f. queynch. but qu.

R.

## R.

R. and its vowel are often transposed. v. Bryddes, brenyng, Crudds, Pomegarnet, &c.

Rapes. 5. Turneps. Lat. *Rapa,* or *Rapum.* vide Junium in voce.

Ryfe. 9 194. Rys, 36. alibi. MS. Ed. 14. Ryys, 192. the Flower, 37. Rice. Fr. Ris. Belg. Rus.

Roo. 14. Roe, the animal.

Rede. 21 alibi. red. A. S. read.

Rooft. 30. alibi. rowfted, 175. fubftantive, 53. to roft. Belg. rooften.

Rether MS Ed 45 a beaft of the horned kind.

Ramme. 33 to fqueeze. but qu.

Renyns 65. perhaps, *rennyng*, i. e. thin, from *renne*, to run. Leland Itin. I p. 5, 6. alibi. Skelton, p. 96. 143. alibi. indeed moft of our old authors. Lel. Coll. IV. p. 287, 288. Chaucer.

Ruayn. v. Chefe

Rape. 83. a difh with no turneps in it Quære if fame c. *Rapil,* Holme III. p. 78. Rapy, MS. Ed. 49.

Refmolle. 96 a difh. v. ad loc.

Ryal 99. *ryalleft* Proem. royal Lel. Coll. IV. p. 250. 257. VI. p 5. bis. 22. Chaucer v Rial.

Rote. 100 Root. *Rotys,* MS. Ed. 32. Chaucer. Junius, v. Root.

Roo Broth. MS. Ed 53.

Roche. 103. the fifh Lel. Coll. VI p 6.

Rygh 105. a fifh. perhaps the Ruffe.

Rawnes. 125. Roes of fifh. *Lye* in Junius. v. Roan.

Reft. MS. Ed. ruftied, of meat. Reftyn, reftyng. N° 57. Ruftinefs Junius. v. Reftie

Rafyols 152. a difh *Ranjoles* Holme III. p. 84.

Reyn MS. Ed 57 Rain. Chaucer.

Ryfhews 182. name of a difh. qu.

Rew de Rumfey. MS. Ed. 44.

[ 151 ]

Ryne hem on a Spyt. 187. run them on a spit.
Rosty. MS. Ed. 44. rost.
Ronde. 196. round. French.
Rosee. 52. a dish. v. ad loc.
Resens. 100. Raysons, 114. Raisins. used of Currants, 14 v. ad loc *Reysons, Reysins.* MS. Ed. II 23. 42. *Rassens* Pottage, is in the second course at archp. Nevill's Feast.

S.

Spine v. Spynee.
Sue forth. 3. et passim. sue. 6. 21. From this short way of writing, and perhaps speaking, we have our *Sewers*, officers of note. and *sewingers*, serving, Lel. Coll. IV. p 291. unless mis-written or misprinted for *shewinge*.
Slype. 11. slip or take off the outer coat. A. S. ſlipan.
Skyrwates 5. 149. Skirrits or Skirwicks.
Savory 6. Sauay. 30. 63. Sawey. 172.
Self. 13. same, made of itself, as self-broth, 22. the owne broth, 122 MS. Ed. 5. 7. Chaucer
Seth. passim MS. Ed. 1, 2. Chaucer. to seeth. A. S. ſeoðan. Seyt. MS. Ed. 1. to strain. 25. 27.
Smite and smyte. 16. 21. 62. cut, hack. A. S. ſmitan.
Sode. v Ysode.
Storchon. MS. Ed. II. 12. v Fitz Stephen. p. 34.
Sum. 20. sumdell, 51. somdel, 171 some, a little, some part. Chaucer has *sum*, and *somdele*. A. S. ſum
Sanders. 20. used for colouring. MS. Ed. 34. v Northumb. Book, p. 415. Sandall wood. The translatois of that very modern book the Arabian Nights Entertainments, frequently have *Sanders* and Sandal wood, as a commodity of the East.
Swyne. 146. alibi. Pork or Bacon. MS. Ed. 3. Bacon, on the contrary, is sometimes used for the animal. Old Plays, II p. 248. Gloss. ad X Script. in v.
See. MS. Ed. 56. Sea. Chaucer.
Sawge 29 *Sauge*, 160 MS Ed 5. Sage. *Pigge en Sage*. E. of Devon's Feast.

Shul.

Shul. 146. fchul. MS. Ed. 4. fhould, as N° 147. fchulle, fchullyn. MS. Ed. 3. 7.

Sawfe Madame. 30. qu. Sauce.

Sandale. MS. Ed. 34.

Sawfe Sarzyne. 84. v. ad loc.

Serpell. 140. wild Thyme. *Serpyllum*.

Sawfe blancke. 136.

Sawfe noyre. 137. 141.

Sawfe verde. 140.

Sow. 30. to few, *fuere*. alfo 175. A. S. ꞅᴉpᴉaṅ.

Stoppe. 34. 48. to ftuff.

Swyng. 39. 43. alibi. MS. Ed. 20. 25. alibi. to fhake, mix. A. S. ꞅꞃenȝan.

Sewe. 20. 29. 40. Sowe. 30. 33. alibi. MS. Ed. 38. Chaucer. Liquor, Broth, Sous. Wiclif. A. S. ꞅeap. v. Lye in 2d alphabet.

Schyms. MS. Ed. 38. Pieces.

Stondyng 45, 46. 7. ftiff, thick.

Smale. 53. alibi. fmall. Lel. Coll. IV. p. 194.

Spynee. 57. v. ad loc.

Straw. 58. ftrew. A. S. ꞅꞇꞃeapᴉan.

Sklyfe. 59. a Slice, or flat Stick for beating any thing. Junius. v. Sclife.

Siryppe. 64. v. ad loc.

Styne. 66. perhaps to clofe. v. yftyned. A. S. ꞇẏnan.

Stere. 67. 145. to ftir. Chaucer. A. S. ꞅꞇẏꞃᴉan.

Sithen. 68. ffithen, 192. then. Chaucer. v. feth and fithe. A. S. ꞅᴉðð an. fithtyn, fethe, feth, fyth. MS. Ed. *then*.

Salat. 76 a Sallad. Saladis, Sallads. Chaucer. Junius, v. *Salad*.

Slete Soppes. 80. flit. A. S. ꞅꞁᴉꞇan.

Spryng. 85. to fprinkle. Wiclif. v. fprenge. A. S. ꞅꞃꞃenȝan.

Samoṅ. 98. Salmon. So Lel. Coll. VI. p. 16, 17. Fr. *Saumon*.

Stepid. 109, 110. fteeped. *Frifius*, ftippen.

[ 153 ]

Sex. 113. 176. Six. A. S.
Sool. 119. *Solys*, 133. Soale, the fish.
Schyl oysters. 121. to shell them. A. S. ꞅcýll, a shell.
Sle. 126. to kill. *Scle*, Chaucer. and *flea*. A. S. ꞅlean.
Sobre Sawſe. 130.
Sowpes. 82. 129. Sops. A S. ꞅop. dorry. MS. Ed. II. 6.
Spell. 140. qu.
Stary. MS. Ed. 32. ſtir.
Swannes. 143. Pye, 79. Cygnets. Lel. Coll. VI. p. 5.
Sonne. MS. Ed. 56. Sun. Chaucer.
Sarſe, and *a Sarſe*. 145. a Sieve or Searſe.
Souple. 152. ſupple. *ſople*, Chaucer; alſo *ſouple*. Fr.
Stewes. 157 170. Liquor. to ſtue, 186. a term well known at this day.
Sais 158. 164. Error perhaps for *Fars*. 167. 169. 172.
Sawcyſter. 160. perhaps, a Sauſſage. from Fr. *Sauciſſe*.
Soler. MS. Ed. 56. a ſolar or upper floor. Chaucer.
Sawgeat. 161. v. ad loc.
Skymō. 162. a Skimmer.
Salwar. 167. v. Calwar.
Sarcyneſs. MS. Ed. 54. v. Sawſe.
Syve, Seve. MS. Ed II. 17, 18. a Sieve. v. Herſyve.
Southrenwode. 172. Southernwood.
Sowie. 173. four. *ſour*, Chaucer.
Stale. 177. Stalk. Handle. uſed now in the North, and elſewhere; as a fork-ſtale; quære a claſis for a fork's tail. Hence, Shaft of an Arrow. Lel. Coll. VI. p. 13. Chaucer. A. S. ꞅtele, or ꞅtela.
Spot. MS. Ed. 57. Sprinkle.
Sachus. 178. a diſh. v. ad loc.
Sachellis. 178 Bags. Satchells.
Spynoches. 180 Spinages. Fr. Eſpinais in plural. but we uſe it in the ſingular. Ital. Spinacchia.
Sit. 192. adhere, and thereby to burn to it. It obtains this ſenſe now in the North, where, after the potage has acquired a moſt diſagreeable taſte by it,

U                         it

it is said to be *pot-fitten*, which in Kent and elsewhere is expreſſed by being *burnt-to*.

Sotiltees. Proem. Suttlety. Lel. Coll. VI. p. 5. ſeq. See Nº 189. There was no grand entertainment without theſe Lel. Coll IV. p. 226, 227. VI. 21. ſeq. made of ſugar and wax. p. 31. and when they were ſerved, or brought in, *at firſt*, they ſeem to have been called *warners*, Lel. Coll. VI. p. 21. 23. VI. p 226, 227 as giving *warning* of the approach of dinner See Notes on Northumb. Book, p. 422, 423. and Mr Pennant's Brit. Zool. p. 496. There are three *ſotiltes* at the E. of Devon's Feaſt, a ſtag, a man, a tree Quere if now ſucceeded by figures of birds, &c. made in lard, and jelly, or in ſugar, to decorate cakes.

Sewyng Proem. following. Leland Coll. IV. p. 293. Chaucer. Fr. *Suivre*.

Spete. MS. Ed. 28. Spit. made of hazel, 58. as Virg. Georg. II. 396.

States. Proem. Perſons.

Scher. MS Ed. 25 ſheer, cut. Chaucer. v. Shere.

Schyveris MS. Ed. 25. II. 27. Shivers. Chaucer. v. Shvere.

Schaw. MS. Ed. 43. ſhave.

## T.

Thurgh. 3. alibi. thorough. A. S. ðuph. *thorw*. MS. Ed. II.

Tanſey. 172. Herb. vide Junii Etymol.

Trape, Trāp. 152. alibi Pan, platter, diſh from Fr.

To gedre. 14. to gydre, 20. to gyder, 39. to gȳd, 53. to gider, 59. to gyd, 111. to gedr, 145. So variouſly is the word *together* here written. A. S. toȝaðepe.

Tredure. 15 name of Cawdel. v. ad loc.

To. 30. 17 MS. Ed. 33. 42. too, and ſo the Saxon. Hence to to. 17. v. ad loc. Alſo, Lel. Coll. IV. p. 181.

p. 181. 206. VI. p. 36. *To* is *till,* MS. Ed. 26. 34. *two.* II. 7. v. Unto.

Thyk. 20. a Verb, to grow thick, as N° 67. thicken taken passively. Adjective, 29. 52. *thik,* 57. *thykke,* 85. *thike,* Chaucer.

Teyse. 20. to pull to pieces with the fingers. v. ad loc. et Junius, voce Tease. Hence teasing for carding wool with teasels, a species of thistle or instrument.

Talbotes. 23. qu v ad loc.

Tat. 30. that. as in Derbysh. *who's tat?* for, who is that? Belg. *dat*

Thenne. 36 alibi. then. Chaucer. A S ðanne.

Thanne. 36. MS. Ed. 25. then. A. S. ðan. than. MS. Ed. 14.

Teer 36. Tear. A. S. tepan.

To fore. 46. alibi. before. Hence our *heretofore.* Wiclif. Chaucer. A. S. topopan.

Thynne 49. MS. Ed. 15. thin A. S. ðinn.

Tailettes. 50. afterwards *Tartletes,* rectiùs ; and so the Contents. *Tortelletti.* Holme. p 85. v. Tartee. Godwin, de Præsul. p. 695. renders *Streblitæ*; et v. Junius, voce Tart.

Thise. 53. alibi. these.

Take. 56. taken. Chaucer.

Thridde. 58. 173. alibi. Third, per metathesin. Chaucer. Thriddendele, 67. Thriddel, 102. 134. *Thredde,* MS. Ed. II. 1. v Junius, voce Thirdendeal.

To done. 68. done. *To* seems to abound, vide Chaucer. v. *To.*

Turnesole. 68. colours *pownas.* vide ad loc.

Ther. 70. 74. they. Chaucer.

Ton tressis. 76. an herb. I amend it to *Ton cressis,* and explain it *Cresses,* being the Saxon tunkenpe, or tuncæpre. See *Lye,* Dict. Sax. Cresses, so as to mean, *one of the Cresses.*

Turbut. 101.

Tried out. 117. drawn out by roasting. See Junius, v. Try.

Tweydel. 124. Twey, MS. Ed. 12. Chaucer. *Twy* for *twae* runs now in the North. A S. τpa, two. bæl, pars, portio.

Talx. 159 Mutton Sewet. v Junii Etym.

Thies, Inyis MS Ed 29, 30 thighs.

Tartes. 164, 165. alibi Tart. de Bry, 166. de Brymlent, 167. tartes of Flesh, 168. of Fish, 170. v. Tarlettes.

Toxh. tough, thick. 173. See Chaucer. v. Tought. A. S τoh.

Tharmys. MS. Ed. 16. Rops, Guts.

There 170. 177 where Chaucer.

Thowche MS. Ed. 48. touch.

To. 185 for Hence, *wherto* is *wherefore*. Chaucer.

Towayl. MS. Ed. II 21. a Towel.

Thee 189 thou, as often now in the North.

Temper. MS. Ed. 1. et sæpe. to mix.

## U.

Uppon. 85. alibi. upon.
Urchon. 176. Urchin, *Erinaceus*.
Unto. MS. Ed. 2. until. v. *To*. Chaucer.

## V.

Violet. 6. v. ad loc.

Verjous. 12. 48. viaws. 154. verious. 15. Verjuice, Fr. Verjus. V. Junium.

Veel. 16. alibi. MS. Ed. 18. Veal.

Vessll. 29. a dish.

Vyne Grace. 61. a mess or dish. *Grees* is the wild Swine. Plott, Hist. of Staff. p. 443. Gloss. to Douglas' Virgil. v. Grisis. and to Chaucer. v. Grys. Thoroton, p. 258. Blount, Tenures. p. 101. *Gresse.*
Lel.

[ 157 ]

Lel. Coll IV. p. 243. *Gres.* 248. Both pork and wine enter into the recipe.

Vyānde Cypre. 97. from the Isle of Cyprus.

Vernage. 132. Vernaccia. a sort of Italian white-wine. In Pref. to *Perlin*, p. xix. mis-written Vervage. See Chaucer. It is a sweet wine in a MS. of Tho. Astle esq. p. 2.

Venyson. 135. often eaten with furmenty, E. of Devon's Feast. *in brothe.* Ibid.

Verde Sawse. 140. it sounds *Green Sauce,* but there is no sorel; sharp, sour Sauce. See Junius, v. Verjuice.

Vervayn. 172.

### W.

Wele. 1. 28. old pronunciation of *well*, now vulgarly used in Derbysh. *wel,* 3. alibi. *wel smale,* 6. very small. v. Lel. Coll. IV. p. 218. 220. Hearne, in Spelm. Life of Ælfred. p. 96.

Wyndewe. 1. winnow. This pronunciation is still retained in Derbyshire, and is not amiss, as the operation is performed by wind. v. omnino, Junius. v. Winnow.

Wayshe, waissh, waische. 1. 5. 17. to wash. A. S. pæɲcan.

Whane, whan. 6. 23 41. when. So Sir Tho. Elliot. v. Britannia. Percy's Songs, I. 77. MS. Romance of Sir Degare versf. 134. A. S. hpænne. wan, wanne. MS. Ed. 25. 38. when.

Wole. Proem. will. *wolt.* 68. wouldst. Chaucer. v. Wol.

Warly, Warliche. 20. 188. gently, warily. A. S. pæpe, wary, prudent. Chaucer. v. Ware, Junius, v. Warie.

Wafrons. 24. Wafers. Junius, v. Wafer.

With

With inne. 30. divifim, for within. So *with oute*, 33.
Welled. 52. v. ad loc. MS. Ed. 23.
Wete. 67. 161. wet, now in the North, and fee Chaucer. A. S. pæt.
Wry. 72. to dry, or cover. Junius, v. Wrie.
Wyn: MS. Ed. 22. alibi. Wine. v. Wyneger.
Wryng thurgh a Straynour. 81. 91. thurgh a cloth, 153. almandes with fair water, 124. wryng out the water. Ibid. wryng parfley up with eggs, 174. Chaucer, voce wrong, ywrong, and wrang. Junius, v. Wring.
Womdes, Wombes. 107. quære the former word ? perhaps being falfely written, it was intended to be obliterated, but forgotten. *Wombes* however means *bellies*, as MS. Ed. 15. See Junius, voce *Womb*.
Wyneger. MS. Ed. 50 Vinegar v. Wyn.
Wone. 107. *a deal* or *quantity*. Chaucer. It has a contrary fenfe though in Junius, v. Whene.
Whete. 116. Wete. MS. Ed. 1. II. 30. Wheat. A. S. hpæte.
Waftel. 118. white Bread. *yfarced*, 159. of it. MS. Ed. 30. II. 18. Gloff. ad X Script. v. Simenellus. Chaucer; where we are referred to Verftegan V. but *Waffel* is explained there, and not *Waftel*; however, fee Stat. 51 Henry III. Hoveden, p. 738. and Junius' Etymol.
Wheyze. 150 171. Whey. A. S. hpæz. Serum Lactis. g often diffolving into y. v. Junium, in Y.
Wynde it to balles. 152. make it into balls, turn it. Chaucer. v Wende. Junius, v. Winde.
Wallenotes. 157 Walnuts. See Junius, in voce.
Wofe of Comfrey. 190. v. ad loc. Juice.
Wex. MS. Ed. 25. Wax.
Were. MS. Ed. 57. where.

Y.

## Y.

Y. is an ufual prefix to adjectives and participles in our old authors. It came from the Saxons; hence ymynced, minced; yflyt, flit, &c. *I* is often fubftituted for it. V. Gloff. to Chaucer, and Lye in Jun. Etym. v. I.

It occurs perpetually for *i*, as ymynced, yflyt, &c. and fo in MS. Editoris alfo.

Written z. 7. 18. alibi. ufed for *gh*, 72. MS. Ed. 33. Chaucer. v. Z. Hence ynouhz, 22. enough. So MS. Ed. paffim. Quere if z is not meant in MSS for g or *t* final.

Dotted, y, after Saxon manner, in MS. Ed. as in Mr. Hearne's edition of Robt. of Gloucefter.

Ycorve. 100, 101. cut in pieces. icorvin, 133. Gloff. to Chaucer. v. *Icorvin*, and *Throtycorve*.

Zelow. 194 *yolow*. MS. Ed. 30. yellow. A. S. zealupe and zelep.

Yolkes. 18. 1 e of eggs. Junius, v. Yelk.

Ygrond. v. Gronden.

Yleefshed. 18. cut it into flices. So, *lefh* it, 65. 67. *leach* is to flice, Holme III. p. 78. or it may mean to *lay in the difh*, 74 81. or diftribute, 85. 117.

Ynouhz 22. ynowh, 23. 28. ynowh, 65. ynow. MS. Ed. 32. Enough. Chaucer has *inough*.

Yfer. 22. 6 i. id eft *ifere*, together. *Feer*, a Companion. Wiclif, in *Feer* and *Scukynge feer*. Chaucer. v. Fere, and Yfere. Junius, v. Yfere.

Yfette. Proem. put down, written.

Yfkaldid. 29. fcalded.

Yfode. 29. *ifode*, 90. *fodden*, 179. boiled. MS. Ed. II. 11. Chaucer. all from to feeth.

Yfope. 30. 63. Yfop. MS. Ed. 53. the herb Hyffop. Chaucer. v. Ifope.

Yforced. v. forced.

Yfafted. 62. qu.

Zif, zyf. MS. Ed. 37. 39. if. also give, II 9. 10.

Ystyned, istyned. 162. 168. to *styne*, 66. seems to mean to close.

Yteyfed. 20. pulled in pieces. v. ad loc. and v. Tcafe.

Ypanced. 62. perhaps pounced, for which see Chaucer.

Yfoñdred. 62. *yfonded*, 97. 102. *yfondyt*, 162. poured, mixed, dissolved. v *found*. Fr. iondu.

Yholes 37. perhaps, hollow.

Ypared. 64. pared.

Ytosted, itosted. 77. 82. toasted.

Iboiled. 114. boiled.

Yest. 151. Junius, v. Yeast.

Igrated. 153. grated.

Ybake. 157. baked.

Ymbre. 100. 165. Ember.

Ypocras. how made, 191. Hippocras. wafers used with it. Lel. Coll. IV. p. 330. VI p. 5, 6. 24. 28. 12. and dry toasts, Rabelais IV. c. 59. *Joly Ypocras*. Lel. Coll. IV. p. 227. VI. p. 22. Bishop Godwin renders it *Vinum aromaticum* It was brought both at beginning of splendid entertainments, if Apicius is to be understood of it. Lib. I. c. 1. See Lister, ad loc and in the middle before the second course; Lel. Coll. IV p. 227. and at the end. It was in use at St. John's Coll. Cambr 50 years ago, and brought in at Christmas at the close of dinner, as anciently most usually it was. It took its name from *Hippocrates' sleeve*, the bag or strainer, through which it was passed. Skinner, v. Claret; and Chaucer or as Junius suggests, because strained *juxta doctrinam Hippocratis*. The Italians call it *hipociasso*. It seems not to have differed much from *Piment*, or Pigment (for which see Chaucer) a rich spiced wine which was sold by Vintners about 1250. Mr. Topham's MS. Hippocras was both white and red. Rabelais, IV. c. 59. and I find it used for sauce to lampreys. Ibid. c. 60.

There

[ 161 ]

There is the procefs at large for making ypocraffe in a MS. of my refpectable Friend Thomas Aftle, efq. p. 2. which we have thought proper to tranfcribe, as follows:

'To make Ypocraffe for lords with gynger,
'fynamon, and graynes fugour, and turefoll: and
'for comyn pepull gynger canell, longe peper, and
'claryffyed hony. Loke ye have feyre pewter
'bafens to kepe in your pouders and your ypocraffe
'to ren ynne. and to vi bafens ye mufte have vi
'renners on a perche as ye may here fee. and loke
'your poudurs and your gynger be redy and well
'paryd or hit be beton in to poud$^r$. Gynger colom-
'byne is the beft gynger, mayken and balandyne
'be not fo good nor holfom.... now thou knowift
'the propertees of Ypocras. Your poudurs muft
'be made everyche by themfelfe, and leid in a bled-
'der in ftore, hange fure your perche with baggs,
'and that no bagge twoyche other, but bafen
'twoyche bafen. The fyrft bagge of a galon, every
'on of the other a potell. Fyrft do in to a bafen a
'galon or ij of redwyne, then put in your pouders,
'and do it in to the renners, and fo in to the feconde
'bagge, then take a pece and aflay it. And yef hit
'be eny thyng to ftronge of gynger alay it withe
'fynamon, and yef it be ftrong of fynamon alay it
'withe fugour cute. And thus fchall ye make per-
'fyte Ypocras And loke your bagges be of boltell
'clothe, and the mouthes opyn, and let it ren in
'v or vi bagges on a perche, and under every bagge
'a clene bafen. The draftes of the fpies is good for
'fewies Put your Ypocrafe in to a ftanche weffell,
'and bynde opon the mouthe a bleddur ftrongly,
'then ferve forthe waffers and Ypocraffe.'

[ 162 ]

## ADDENDA.

p. i. add at bottom. ' vi. 22. where *Noah* and the
' beasts are to live on the same food '

xiv. after *ingeniosa gula est*, add, ' The *Italians* now
' eat many things which we think perfect carrion.
' *Ray*, Trav. p. 362. 406. The *French* eat frogs
' and snails. The *Tartars* feast on horse-flesh, the
' *Chinese* on dogs, and meer *Savages* eat every
' thing *Goldsmith*, Hist. of the Earth, &c. II. p. 347,
' 348. 395. III p. 297. IV. p. 112. 121, &c.'

xviii. lin. 1. after *ninth Iliad*, add, ' And Dr. *Shaw*
' writes, p. 301, that even now in the East, the
' greatest prince is not ashamed to fetch a lamb
' from his herd and kill it, whilst the princess is
' impatient till she hath prepared her fire and her
' kettle to dress it.'

Ibid. lin. 12. after *heretofore* add, ' we have some
' good families in England of the name of *Cook* or
' *Cole*. I know not what they may think; but we
' may depend upon it, they all originally sprang
' from real and professional cooks, and they need
' not be ashamed of their extraction, any more
' than the *Butlers, Packers, Spencers*, &c.'

xix. add at bottom, ' reflect on the *Spanish Olio* or
' *Olla podrida*, and the French fricassée.'

xxi. lin ult *intended*. add, ' See *Ray*, Trav p. 283.
' 207. and *Knight's* Trav p. 112.'

ADVER-

## ADVERTISEMENT.

SINCE the foregoing sheets were printed off, the following very curious Rolls have happily fallen into the Editor's hand, by the favour of John Charles Brooke, Esq. Somerset Herald. They are extracted from a MS. belonging to the family of Nevile of Chevet, near Wakefield, com. Ebor. and thence copied, under the direction of the Rev. Richard Kay, D. D. Prebendary of Durham.

These Rolls are so intimately connected with our subject, as exhibiting the dishes of which our Roll of *Cury* teaches the dressing and preparation, that they must necessarily be deemed a proper appendix to it. They are moreover amusing, if not useful, in another respect, *viz.* as exhibiting the gradual prices of provisions, from the dates of our more ancient lists, and the time when these Rolls were composed, in the reign of Henry VIII. For the further illustration of this subject, an extract from the old Account-Book of *Luton*, 19 *Hen.* VIII. is super-added; where the prices of things in the South, at the same period, may be feen. And whoever pleafes to go further into this matter of *prices*, may compare them with the particulars and expence of a dinner at Stationer's-Hall, A.D 1556. which appeared in the St. James's Chronicle of April 22, 1780.

We cannot help thinking that, upon all accounts, the additions here prefented to our friends muft needs prove exceedingly acceptable to them.

ROLLS

# ROLLS OF PROVISIONS,

With their PRICES, DISHES, &c.

Temp. H. VIII.

THE marriage of my fon-in-law [a] Gervas Clifton and my daughter Mary Nevile, the 17th day of January, in the 21ft year of the reigne of our Soveraigne Lord King Henry the VIIIth.

|  | £. | s. | d. |
|---|---|---|---|
| Firft, for the apparell of the faid Gervys Clifton and Mary Nevill, 21 yards of Ruffet Damafk, every yard 8 s [b], | 7 | 14 | 8 |
| Item, 6 yards of White Damafk, every yard 8 s. |  | 48 | 0 |

---

[a] Gervas] below *Gervyys*. So unfettled was our orthography, even in the reign of Henry VIII So *Nevile*, and below *Nevill*. Mary, third daughter of Sir John Nevil of Chevet, was firft wife of Sir Gerv. Clifton of Clifton, com Nott Knight.

[b] 8 s.] The fum is £ 7. 14 s. 8 d but ought to be £ 8 8 s. fo that there is fome miftake here. N B This tranfcript is given in our common figures, but the original, no coubt, is in the Roman.

|   |   £. | s. | d. |
|---|---|---|---|
| Item, 12 yards of Tawney Camlet, every yard 2s. 8d ᶜ. |   | 49 | 4 |
| Item, 6 yards of Tawney Velvet, every yard 14s. |   | 4 | 4 | 0 |
| Item, 2 Rolls of Buckrom, | 0 | 6 | 0 |
| Item, 3 Black Velvet Bonnits for women, every bonnit 17s. |   | 51 | 0 |
| Item, a Fronflet ᵈ of Blue Velvet, | 0 | 7 | 6 |
| Item, an ounce of Damask Gold ᵉ, | 0 | 4 | 0 |
| Item, 4 Laynes ᶠ of Frontlets, | 0 | 2 | 8 |
| Item, an Eyye ᵍ of Pearl, |   | 24 | 0 |
| Item, 3 pair of Gloves, | 0 | 2 | 10 |
| Item, 3 yards of Kerfey; 2 black, 1 white, | 0 | 7 | 0 |
| Item, Lining for the fame, | 0 | 2 | 0 |
| Item, 3 Boxes to carry bonnits in, | 0 | 1 | 0 |
| Item, 3 Pafts ʰ, | 0 | 0 | 9 |
| Item, a Furr of White Lufants ⁱ, |   | 40 | 0 |
| Item, 12 Whit Heares ᵏ, |   | 12 | 0 |
| Item, 20 Black Conies, |   | 10 | 0 |

ᶜ 2s. 8d.] This again is wrongly computed There may be other miftakes of the fame kind, which is here noted once for all, the reader will eafily rectify them himfelf.

ᵈ Fronflet.] f. Frontlet, as lin. 10.

ᵉ Damask Gold ] Gold of Damafcus, perhaps for powder.

ᶠ Laynes.] qu.

ᵍ Eyye.] f Egg.

ʰ Pafts.] Paftboards.

ⁱ Lufants.] qu

ᵏ Heares]. f. Hares.

Item,

|  | £. | s. | d. |
|---|---|---|---|
| Item, A pair of Myllen [1] Sleves of white fattin, | 0 | 8 | 0 |
| Item, 30 White Lamb Skins, | 0 | 4 | 0 |
| Item, 6 yards of White Cotton, | 0 | 3 | 0 |
| Item, 2 yards and ½ black fattin, | 0 | 14 | 9 |
| Item, 2 Girdles, | 0 | 5 | 4 |
| Item, 2 ells of White Ribon, for tippets, | 0 | 1 | 1 |
| Item, an ell of Blue Sattin, | 0 | 6 | 8 |
| Item, a Wedding Ring of Gold, | 0 | 12 | 4 |
| Item, a Millen Bonnit, dreffed with Agletts, | 0 | 11 | 0 |
| Item, a yard of right White Sattin, | 0 | 12 | 0 |
| Item, a yard of White Sattin of Bridge [m], | 0 | 2 | 4 |

The Expence of the Dinner, at the marriage of faid Gervys Clifton and Mary Nevile. Imprimis,

|  |  |  |  |
|---|---|---|---|
| Three Hogfheads of Wine, 1 white, 1 red, 1 claret, | 5 | 5 | 0 |
| Item, 2 Oxen, | 3 | 0 | 0 |
| Item, 2 Brawns [n], | 1 | 0 | 0 |
| Item, 2 Swans [o], every Swan 2s, | 0 | 12 | 0 |

---

[1] Myllen]. *Milan*, city of Lombardy, whence our *millaner*, now *milliner*, written below *millen*.

[m] Bridge]. Brugge, or Bruges, in Flanders.

[n] Brawns] The Boar is now called a Brawn in the North, vid. p. 126.

[o] 2 Swans]. f. 6 Swans.

[ 168 ]

|  | £. | s. | d. |
|---|---|---|---|
| Item, 9 Cranes<sup>p</sup>, every Crane 3 s. 4 d. | 1 | 10 | 0 |
| Item, 16 Heron fews<sup>q</sup>, every one 12 d. | 0 | 16 | 0 |
| Item, 10 Bitterns, each 14d. | 0 | 11 | 8 |
| Item, 60 couple of Conies, every couple 5d, | | 25 | 0 |
| Item, as much Wild-fowl, and the charge of the fame, as coft | 3 | 6 | 8 |
| Item, 16 Capons of Greafe<sup>r</sup>, | 0 | 16 | 0 |
| Item, 30 other Capons, | 0 | 15 | 0 |
| Item, 10 Pigs, every one 5d. | 0 | 4 | 2 |
| Item, 6 Calves, | 0 | 16 | 0 |
| Item, 1 other Calf, | 0 | 3 | 0 |
| Item, 7 Lambs, | 0 | 10 | 0 |
| Item, 6 Withers<sup>s</sup>, every Wither 2s. 4d. | 0 | 14 | 0 |
| Item, 8 Quarters of Barley<sup>t</sup> Malt, every quarter 14s. | 5 | 10 | 0 |
| Item, 3 Quarters of Wheat, every quarter 18 s. | | 54 | 0 |
| Item, 4 dozen of Chickens, | 0 | 6 | 0 |

Befides Butter, Eggs, Verjuice, and Vinegar.

---

<sup>p</sup> Cranes] v. p 67.

<sup>q</sup> Heron fews] In one word, rather. See p 139.

<sup>r</sup> of Greafe ] I prefume fatted.

<sup>s</sup> Withers]. Weathers.

<sup>t</sup> Barley malt] So diftinguifhed, becaufe wheat and oats were at this time fometime malted. See below, p 172.

In

[ 169 ]

### In Spices as followeth.

|  | £. | s. | d. |
|---|---|---|---|
| Two Loaves of Sugar [u], weighing 16 lb. 12 oz. at 7 d. per lb. | 0 | 9 | 9 |
| Item, 6 pound of Pepper, every pound 22 d. | 0 | 11 | 0 |
| Item, 1 pound of Ginger, | 0 | 2 | 4 |
| Item, 12 pound of Currants, every pound 3½ d. | 0 | 3 | 6 |
| Item, 12 lb of Proynes [x], every pound 2 d. | 0 | 2 | 0 |
| Item, 2 lb. of Marmalet, | 0 | 2 | 1 |
| Item, 2 [y] Poils of Sturgeon, | 0 | 12 | 4 |
| Item, a Barrel for the same, | 0 | 0 | 6 |
| Item, 12 lb. of Dates, every lb. 4 d. | 0 | 4 | 0 |
| Item. 12 lb. of Great Raisons [z], | 0 | 2 | 0 |
| Item, 1 lb. of Cloves and Mace, | 0 | 8 | 0 |
| Item, 1 quarter of Saffron, | 0 | 4 | 0 |
| Item, 1 lb. of Tornself [a], | 0 | 4 | 0 |
| Item, 1 lb of Ising-glass, | 0 | 4 | 0 |
| Item, 1 lb. of Biskitts, | 0 | 1 | 0 |
| Item, 1 lb. of Carraway Seeds, | 0 | 1 | 0 |
| Item, 2 lb. of Cumfitts, | 0 | 2 | 0 |
| Item, 2 lb. of Torts [b] of Portugal, | 0 | 2 | 0 |

[u] Loaves of Sugar]. So that they had now a method of refining it, v p xxvi.

[x] Proynes]. Prunes, v p. 148.

[y] Poils] Misread, perhaps, for Joils, i. e. Jowls.

[z] Great Raisons,] v p. 38.

[a] Tornself] Turnsole, v. p. 38.

[b] Torts]. qu.

|  | £. | s. | d. |
|---|---|---|---|
| Item, 4 lb. of Liquorice and Annifeeds, | 0 | 1 | 0 |
| Item, 3 lb. of Green Ginger, | 0 | 4 | 0 |
| Item, 3 lb. of Suckets [c], | 0 | 4 | 0 |
| Item, 3 lb. of Orange Buds, 4s. | 0 | 5 | 4 |
| Item, 4 lb. of Oranges in Syrup, | 0 | 5 | 4 |
| Totall £. | 61 | 8 | 8 |

[c] Suckets]. Thefe, it feems, were fold ready prepared in the fhops. See the following Rolls.

Sir John Nevile, ⎫ The marriage of my Son in-law,
of Chete, Knight. ⎭ Roger Rockley[a], and my daughter Elizabeth Nevile, the 14th of January, in the 17th year of the reigne of our Soveraigne Lord King Henry the VIIIth.

|  | £. | s. | d. |
|---|---|---|---|
| First, for the expence of their Apparel, 22 yards of Russet Sattin, at 8s. per yard, | 8 | 16 | 0 |
| Item, 2 Mantilles of Skins, for his gown, |  | 48 | 0 |
| Item, 2 yards and ½ of black velvet, for his gown, | 0 | 30 | 0 |
| Item, 9 yards of Black Sattin, for his Jacket and Doublet, at 8s. the yard, | 3 | 12 | 0 |
| Item, 7 yards of Black Sattin, for her Kertill, at 8s. per yard, |  | 56 | 0 |
| Item, a Roll of Buckrom, | 0 | 2 | 8 |
| Item, a Bonnit of Black Velvet, | 0 | 15 | 0 |
| Item, a Frontlet for the same Bonnit, | 0 | 12 | 0 |
| Item, for her Smock, | 0 | 5 | 0 |
| Item, for a pair of perfumed Gloves, | 0 | 3 | 4 |
| Item, for a pair of other Gloves, | 0 | 0 | 4 |

[a] Rockley] Elizabeth eldest daughter of Sir John Nevile, married, Roger eldest son, and afterwards heir, of Sir Thomas Rockley of Rockley, in the parish of Worsborough, Knight.

## Second Day.

|  | £. | s. | d. |
|---|---|---|---|
| Item, for 22 yards of Tawney Camlet, at 2s. 4d. per yard, | | 51 | 4 |
| Item, 3 yards of Black Sattin, for lining her gown, at 8s per yard, | | 24 | 0 |
| Item, 2 yards of Black Velvet, for her gown, | | 30 | 0 |
| Item, a Roll of Buckrom, for her Gown, | 0 | 2 | 8 |
| Item, 7 yards of Yellow Sattin Bridge[b], at 2s. 4d. per yard, | | 26 | 4 |
| Item, for a pair of Hose, | 0 | 2 | 4 |
| Item, for a pair Shoes, | 0 | 1 | 4 |
| Sum £. | 27 | 8 | 0 |

Item, for Dinner, and the Expence of the said Marriage of Roger Rockley, and the said Elizabeth Nevile.

|  | £. | s. | d. |
|---|---|---|---|
| Imprimis, eight quarters of Barley-malt, at 10s. per quarter, | 4 | 0 | 0 |
| Item, 3 quarters and ½ of Wheat, at 14s. 4d. per quarter, | | 56 | 8 |
| Item, 2 Hogsheads of Wine, at 40s. | 4 | 0 | 0 |
| Item, 1 Hogshead of Red Wine, at | 0 | 40 | 0 |
| Sum Total £ | 39 | 8 | 0 |

[b] Br*i*dge]. See above, p. 167, note [m].

For

For the First Course at Dinner.

Imprimis, Brawn with Musterd, served alone with Malmsey.
Item, Frumety [c] to Pottage.
Item, a Roe roasted for Standert [d].
Item, Peacocks, 2 of a Dish.
Item, Swans 2 of a Dish.
Item, a great Pike in a Dish.
Item, Conies roasted 4 of a Dish.
Item, Venison roasted.
Item, Capon of Grease, 3 of a Dish.
Item, Mallards [e], 4 of Dish.
Item, Teals, 7 of a Dish.
Item, Pyes baken [f], with Rabbits in them.
Item, Baken Orange.
Item, a Flampett [g].
Item, Stoke Fritters [h].
Item, Dulcets [i], ten of Dish.
Item, a Tart.

[c] Frumety]. v. p 135.
[d] Standert]. A large or standing dish. See p. 174. l. 3.
[e] Mallards]. v p 144
[f] Baken] baked.
[g] Flampett]. f. Flaunpett, or Flaumpeyn, v p. 136.
[h] Stoke Fritters]. Baked on a hot-iron, used still by the Brewers, called a stoker.
[i] Dulcets]. qu.

## Second Course.

First, Marterns [k] to Pottage.
Item for a Standert, Cranes 2 of a dish.
Item, Young Lamb, whole roasted.
Item, Great Fresh Sammon Gollis [l].
Item, Heron Sues, 3 of a dish.
Item, Bitterns, 3 of a dish.
Item, Pheasants, 4 of a dish.
Item, a Great Sturgeon Poil.
Item, Partridges, 8 of a dish.
Item, Plover, 8 of a dish.
Item, Stints [m], 8 of a dish.
Item, Curlews [n], 3 of a dish.
Item, a whole Roe, baken.
Item, Venison baken, red and fallow [o].
Item, a Tart.
Item, a March [p] Payne.
Item, Gingerbread.
Item, Apples and Cheese scraped with Sugar and Sage.

[k] Marterns] qu. it is written Martens, below.

[l] Gollis] f. Jowls

[m] Stints]. The Stint, or Purre, is one of the Sandpipers. Pennant, Brit Zool, II 374.

[n] Curlews] See above, p. 130 and below. Curlew Knaves, also below.

[o] Fallow ] If I remember right, Dr Goldsmith says, Fallow-deer were brought to us by King James I. but see again below, more than once

[p] March Payne] A kind of Cake, very common long after this time, v. below.

For

## For Night.

First a Play, and straight after the play a Mask, and when the Mask was done then the Banckett [a], which was 110 dishes, and all of meat, and then all the Gentilmen and Ladys danced, and this continued from the Sunday to the Saturday afternoon.

The Expence in the Week for Flesh and Fish for the same marriage.

|  | £. | s. | d. |
|---|---|---|---|
| Imprimis, 2 Oxen, | 3 | 0 | 0 |
| Item, 2 Brawns, |  | 22 | 0 |
| Item, 2 Roes 10s. and for servants going, 5s. | 0 | 15 | 0 |
| Item, in Swans, | 0 | 15 | 0 |
| Item, in Cranes 9, |  | 30 | 0 |
| Item, in Peacocks 12, | 0 | 16 | 0 |
| Item, in Great Pike, for flesh dinner, 6, |  | 30 | 0 |
| Item, in Conies, 21 dozen, | 5 | 5 | 0 |
| Item, in Venison, Red Deer Hinds 3, and fetching them, | 0 | 10 | 0 |
| Item, Fallow Deer Does 12, | — | — | — |
| Item, Capons of Grease 72, | 3 | 12 | 0 |
| Item, Mallards and Teal, 30 dozen, | 3 | 11 | 8 |
| Item, Lamb 3, | 0 | 4 | 0 |
| Item, Heron Sues, 2 doz. |  | 24 | 0 |

[a] Banckett]. Banquet.

|  |  | £. | s. | d. |
|---|---|---:|---:|---:|
| Item, Shovelords ʳ, 2 doz. |  |  | 24 | 0 |
| Item, in Bytters ˢ 12, |  |  | 16 | 0 |
| Item, in Pheasants 18, |  |  | 24 | 0 |
| Item, in Partridges 40, |  | 0 | 6 | 8 |
| Item, in Curlews 18, |  |  | 24 | 0 |
| Item, in Plover, 3 dozen, |  | 0 | 5 | 0 |
| Item, in Stints, 5 doz. |  | 0 | 9 | 0 |
| Item, in Sturgeon, 1 Goyle ᵗ, |  | 0 | 5 | 0 |
| Item, 1 Seal ᵘ, |  | 0 | 13 | 4 |
| Item, 1 Porpose ˣ, |  | 0 | 13 | 4 |

£.

### For Frydays and Saturdays.

First, Leich Brayne ʸ.
Item, Frometye Pottage.

---

ʳ Shovelords] Shovelers, a species of the Wild Duck. Shovelards, below.

ˢ Bytters]. Bitterns, above; but it is often written without n, as below

ᵗ Goyle]. Jowl, v. above, p. 174 l 5.

ᵘ Seal]. One of those things not eaten now, but see p. 147 above, and below, p. 180 l 6

ˣ Porpose] v p 147, above.

ʸ Leich Brayne]. v. p. 141, above but qu. as to Brayne.

Item,

Item, Whole Ling and Huberdyne [z].
Item, Great Goils [a] of Salt Sammon.
Item, Great Salt Eels.
Item, Great Salt Sturgeon Goils.
Item, Fresh Ling.
Item, Fresh Turbut.
Item, Great Pike [b].
Itdm, Great Goils of Fresh Sammon.
Item, Great Ruds [c].
Item, Baken Turbuts.
Item, Tarts of 3 several meats [d].

## Second Course.

First, Martens to Pottage.
Item, a Great Fresh Sturgeon Goil.
Item, Fresh Eel roasted.
Item, Great Brett.
Item, Sammon Chines broil'd.
Item, Roasted Eels.
Item, Roasted Lampreys.
Item, Roasted Lamprons [e].
Item, Great Burbutts [f].

[z] Huberdyne]. miswritten for Haberdine, i. e. from Aberdeen; written below Heberdine.

[a] Goils] v. above, p. 174. l. 5.

[b] Pyke]. v. above, p 50. and below, often.

[c] Ruds]. qu. Roaches, v below.

[d] meats]. Viands, but not Fleshmeats.

[e] Lamprons] v. p. 142, above.

[f] Burbatts]. qu. Turbuts.

Item,

Item, Sammon baken.
Item, Fresh Eel baken.
Item, Fresh Lampreys, baken.
Item, Clear Jilly [g].
Item, Gingerbread.

Waiters at the said Marriage.

Storrers, Carver.
Mr. Henry Nevile, Sewer.
Mr. Thomas Drax, Cupbearer.
Mr. George Pashlew, for the Sewer board end.
John Merys,  } Marshalls.
John Mitchill, }
Robert Smallpage, for the Cupboard.
William Page, for the Celler.
William Barker, for the Ewer.
Robett Sike the Younger, and
John Hiperon, for Butterye.

To wait in the Parlour.

Richard Thornton.
Edmund North.
Robert Sike the Elder.
William Longley.
Robert Live.
William Cook.
Sir John Burton, Steward.
My brother Stapleton's servant.
My son Rockley's servant to serve in the state.

[g] Jilly]. Jelly.

[ 179 ]

The Charges of Sir John Nevile, of Chete, Knight, being Sheriff of Yorkshire in the 19th year of the reigne of King Henry VIII.

Lent Assizes.

|  | £. | s. | d. |
|---|---|---|---|
| Imprimis, in Wheat 8 quarters, | 8 | 0 | 0 |
| Item, in Malt, 11 quarters, | 7 | 6 | 8 |
| Item, in Beans, 4 quarters, | 3 | 4 | 0 |
| Item, in Hay, 6 loads, |  | 25 | 0 |
| Item, in Litter, 2 loads, | 0 | 4 | 0 |
| Item, part of the Judge's Horses in the inn, | 0 | 13 | 4 |
| Item, 5 hogsheads of Wine, 3 claret, 1 white, 1 red, | 10 | 16 | 4 |
| Item, Salt Fish, 76 couple, | 3 | 16 | 4 |
| Item, 2 barrells Herrings, |  | 25 | 6 |
| Item, 2 Barrells Salmon, | 3 | 1 | 0 |
| Item, 12 seams [a] of Sea Fish, | 6 | 4 | 0 |
| Item, in Great Pike and Pickering, 6 score and 8, | 8 | 0 | 0 |
| Item, 12 Great Pike from Ramsay, | 2 | 0 | 0 |
| Item, in Pickerings from Holdess IIII xx, | 3 | 0 | 0 |
| Item, Received of Rythei 20 great Breams, |  | 20 | 0 |
| Item, Received of said Ryther, 12 great Tenches, | 0 | 16 | 0 |

[a] seams]. quarter, much used in Kent, v. infra.

[ 180 ]

|  | £. | s. | d. |
|---|---|---|---|
| Item, Received of said Ryther 12 great Eels and 106 Touling [b] Eels, and 200 lb. of Brewit [c] Eels, and 20 great Ruds, | | 40 | 0 |
| Item, in great Fresh Sammon, 28 | 3 | 16 | 8 |
| Item, a Barrell of Sturgeon, | | 46 | 8 |
| Item, a Firkin of Seal, | 0 | 16 | 8 |
| Item, a little barrell of Syrope [d], | 0 | 6 | 8 |
| Item, 2 barrells of all manner of Spices, | 4 | 10 | 0 |
| Item, 1 bag of Isinglass, | 0 | 3 | 0 |
| Item, a little barrell of Oranges, | 0 | 4 | 0 |
| Item, 24 gallons of Malmsey, | 0 | 16 | 0 |
| Item, 2 little barrells of Green Ginger and Suckets, | 0 | 3 | 0 |
| Item, 3 Bretts, | 0 | 12 | 0 |
| Item, in Vinegar, 13 gallon, 1 quart | 0 | 6 | 8 |
| Item, 8 large Table Cloths of 8 yards in length, 7 of them 12 d per yard, and one 16 d, | 3 | 6 | 8 |
| Item, 6 doz. Manchetts [e], | 0 | 6 | 0 |
| Item, 6 gallons Vergis [f], | 0 | 4 | 8 |
| Item, in Mayne Bread [g], | 0 | 0 | 8 |

[b] Touling Eels] qu see below.

[c] Brewit Eels]. *i. e.* for Brewet, for which see above, p. 127. also here, below

[d] Syrope] v. p. 36. above.

[e] Manchetts]. a species of Bread, see below.

[f] Vergis]. Verjuice.

[g] Mayne Bread]. Pain du main, v. p 147 above

Item

[ 181 ]

|  | £. | s. | d. |
|---|---|---|---|
| Item, bread bought for March Payne, | 0 | 0 | 8 |
| Item, for Sugar and Almonds, besides the 2 barrels, | 0 | 11 | 0 |
| Item, for Salt | 0 | 6 | 0 |
| Item, for 5 gallons of Muſtard, | 0 | 2 | 6 |
| Item, a Draught of Fiſh, 2 great Pikes and 200 Breams, | 0 | 26 | 8 |
| Item, 3 gallons of Honey, | 0 | 3 | 9 |
| Item, 6 Horſe-loads of Charcoal, | 0 | 2 | 8 |
| Item, 3 Load of Talwood [h] and Bavings, | 0 | 3 | 4 |
| Item, 4 Streyners, | 0 | 1 | 0 |
| Item, for Graines [i], | 0 | 0 | 4 |
| Item, 20 doz. of Cups, | 0 | 6 | 8 |
| Item, 6 Flaſkits and 1 Maund [k], | 0 | 3 | 4 |
| Item, 1 doz Earthen Potts, | 0 | 0 | 6 |
| Item, 2 Staff Torches, | 0 | 4 | 0 |
| Item, for Yearbes [l], 5 days, | 0 | 1 | 8 |
| Item, for Waferans, 5 days [m], | 0 | 1 | 8 |
| Item, for Onions, | 0 | 1 | 0 |

[h] Talwood and Bavings]. Chord-wood, and Bavins. See Dr Birch's Life of Prince Henry Wetwood and Bevins occur below, p 184.

[i] Grains]. qu.

[k] Maund]. a large Baſket, now uſed for Apples, &c

[l] Yearbes] yerbs are often pronounced ſo now, whence *Yerby Greaſe*, for Herb of Grace.

[m] 5 days] qu perhaps gathering, or fetching them,

|  | £. | s. | d. |
|---|---|---|---|
| Item, 2 Gallipots, | 0 | 0 | 8 |
| Item, for Yeast, 5 days, | 0 | 1 | 8 |
| Item, 20 doz. borrowed Vessels, | 0 | 5 | 1 |
| Item, for Carriage of Wheat, Malt, Wine, and Wood, from the Water-side, | 0 | 15 | 0 |
| Item, for Parker the Cook, and other Cooks and Water-bearers, | 4 | 10 | 0 |
| Item, 6 doz. of Trenchers, | 0 | 0 | 4 |
| First, for making a Cupboard, | 0 | 1 | 4 |

---

ᵃ Waferans] v. above, p 157.

The Charge of the said Sir John Nevile of Chete at Lammas Assizes, in the 20th Year of the Reign of King Henry the VIIIth.

|  | £. | s. | d. |
|---|---|---|---|
| Imprimis, in Wheat, 9 quarters, | 12 | 0 | 0 |
| Item, in Malt, 12 quarters, | 10 | 0 | 0 |
| Item, 5 Oxen, | 6 | 13 | 4 |
| Item, 24 Weathers, | 3 | 4 | 0 |
| Item, 6 Calves, |  | 20 | 0 |
| Item, 60 Capons of Grease, |  | 25 | 0 |
| Item, other Capons, | 3 | 14 | 0 |
| Item, 24 Pigs, | 0 | 14 | 0 |
| Item, 3 hogsheads of Wine, | 8 | 11 | 8 |
| Item, 22 Swans, | 5 | 10 | 0 |
| Item, 12 Cranes, | 4 | 0 | 0 |
| Item, 30 Heronsews, |  | 30 | 0 |
| Item, 12 Shovelards, |  | 12 | 0 |
| Item, 10 Bitters, |  | 13 | 4 |
| Item, 80 Partridges, |  | 26 | 8 |
| Item, 12 Pheasants, |  | 20 | 0 |
| Item, 20 Curlews, |  | 26 | 8 |
| Item, Curlew Knaves 32, |  | 32 | 0 |
| Item, 6 doz. Plovers, | 0 | 12 | 0 |
| Item, 30 doz. Pidgeons, | 0 | 7 | 6 |
| Item, Mallards, Teal, and other Wild Fowl, |  | 42 | 0 |
| Item, 2 Baskets of all manner of Spice, | 5 | 0 | 0 |

[ 184 ]

|  | £. | s. | d. |
|---|---|---|---|
| Item, in Malmsey, 24 Gallons, |  | 32 | 0 |
| Item, in Bucks, | 10 | 0 | 0 |
| Item, in Stags, | — | — | — |

### Fryday and Saturday.

|  | £. | s. | d. |
|---|---|---|---|
| First, 3 couple of great Ling, |  | 12 | 0 |
| Item, 40 couple of Heberdine, |  | 40 | 0 |
| Item, Salt Sammon, |  | 20 | 0 |
| Item, Fresh Sammon and Great, | 3 | 6 | 8 |
| Item, 6 great Pike, |  | 12 | 0 |
| Item, 80 Pickerings, | 4 | 0 | 0 |
| Item, 300 great Breams, | 15 | 0 | 0 |
| Item, 40 Tenches, |  | 26 | 8 |
| Item, 80 Tooling Eels and Brevet Eels, and 15 Ruds, |  | 32 | 0 |
| Item, a Firkin of Sturgeon, |  | 16 | 0 |
| Item, in Fresh Seals, |  | 13 | 4 |
| Item, 8 seame of Fresh Fish, | 4 | 0 | 0 |
| Item, 2 Bretts, |  | 8 | 0 |
| Item, a barrell of Green Ginger and Sucketts, |  | 4 | 0 |
| Item, 14 gallon of Vinegar, |  | 7 | 7½ |
| Item, 6 horse-loads of Charcoal, |  | 2 | 4 |
| Item, 40 load of Wetwood and Bevins, |  | 53 | 4 |
| Item, for Salt, |  | 5 | 2 |
| Item, 6 doz of Manchetts, |  | 6 | 0 |
| Item, Gingerbread for March Payne, |  | 0 | 8 |
| Item, 5 gallon of Mustard, |  | 2 | 6 |

Item,

|  | £. | s. | d. |
|---|---|---|---|
| Item, for loan of 6 doz. veffels, |  | 5 | 2 |
| Item, 3 gallons of Honey, |  | 3 | 9 |
| Item, for the cofts of Cooks and Water-bearers, | 4 | 0 | 0 |
| Item, for the Judges and Clerks of the Affize, for their Horfe-meat in the Inn, and for their Houfekeeper's meat, and the Clerk of the Affize Fee, | 10 | 0 | 0 |
| Item, for my Livery Coats, embroidered, | 50 | 0 | 0 |
| Item, for my Horfes Provender, Hay, Litter, and Grafs, at both the Affizes, | 6 | 13 | 4 |

[ 186 ]

In a vellum MS. Account-Book of the Gild of the Holy Trinity at Luton, com. Bedford, from 19 Hen. VIII. to the beginning of Ed. VI. there are the expences of their Anniverſary Feaſts, from year to year, exhibiting the ſeveral Proviſions, with their prices. The feaſt of 19 Hen. VIII. is hereunder inſerted; from whence ſome judgement may be formed of the reſt.

|  | £. | s. | d. |
|---|---:|---:|---:|
| 5 quarters, 6 buſhels of Wheat, |  | 50 | 2 |
| 3 buſhels Wheat Flower, | 0 | 5 | 11 |
| 6 quarters malte, |  | 29 | 0 |
| 72 Barrels Beer, | 0 | 12 | 10 |
| Brewing 6 quarters Malte, | 0 | 4 | 0 |
| Bakyng, | 0 | 1 | 6 |
| 82 Geys, | 1 | 0 | 7 |
| 47 Pyggs, | 1 | 3 | 10 |
| 64 Capons, | 1 | 9 | 8½ |
| 74 Chekyns, | 0 | 8 | 2 |
| 84 Rabetts, and Carriage, | 0 | 10 | 8 |
| Beyf, |  |  |  |
| 4 quarters, | 1 | 0 | 0 |
| a Lyfte, | 0 | 0 | 8 |
| a Shodour & Cromys, | 0 | 0 | 11 |

Moton

|                                      | £. | s. | d.   |
|--------------------------------------|----|----|------|
| Moton & Welle [a].                   |    |    |      |
| 1 quarter,                           | 0  | 0  | 8    |
| 2 leggs of Welle & 2 Shodours,       | 0  | 1  | 0    |
| A Marebone & Suet, & 3 Calwisfere,   | 0  | 0  | 4    |
| 1 quarter of Moton, and 6 Calwisfere,| 0  | 0  | 9    |
| 20 Lamys,                            | 1  | 5  | 10   |
| Dreffyng of Lamys,                   | 0  | 0  | 6    |
| Wine, 2 galons, a potell, & a pynte, | 0  | 1  | 9    |
| Wenegar 3 potellis,                  | 0  | 1  | 0    |
| Warg [b] 1 galon,                    | 0  | 0  | 2½   |
| Spyce,                               |    |    |      |
| 3 lb Pepur & half,                   | 0  | 6  | 11   |
| 4 oz. of Clovis & Mace, & quartron,  | 0  | 3  | 4    |
| 11 lb. of Sugur & half,              | 0  | 7  | 0    |
| ½ lb. of Sinamon,                    | 0  | 3  | 4    |
| 12 lb. of gret Refons,               | 0  | 1  | 0    |
| 6 lb. of fmale Refons,               | 0  | 1  | 4    |
| ½ lb. of Gynger,                     | 0  | 1  | 10   |
| ½ lb. of Sandurs,                    | 0  | 0  | 8    |
| 1 lb. of Lycoras,                    | 0  | 0  | 6    |
| 4 lb. of Prunys,                     | 0  | 0  | 8    |
| 1 lb. of Comfetts,                   | 0  | 0  | 8    |
| ½ lb. of Turnefell,                  | 0  | 0  | 3    |
| 1 lb. of Grenys,                     | 0  | 1  | 9    |
| 1 lb. of Aneffeds,                   | 0  | 0  | 5    |

[a] Veal, now in the South pronounced with *W*.
[b] Verjuice.

2 lb.

|  | £. | s. | d. |
|---|---|---|---|
| 2 lb of Almonds, | 0 | 0 | 5 |
| 2 oz. of Safron and a quartron, | 0 | 2 | 9 |
| 2 lb. of Dats, | 0 | 0 | 8 |
| Eggs 600, | 0 | 6 | 0 |
| Butter, | 0 | 2 | 7 |
| Mylke 19 galons, | 0 | 1 | 7 |
| 8 galons and 2 gal. of Crem, | 0 | 1 | 3½ |
| Hone 2 galons, | 0 | 3 | 0 |
| Salte ½ boshell, | 0 | 0 | 8 |
| Fyshe, |  |  |  |
| Fresche, and the careeg from London, | 0 | 3 | 8 |
| A fresche Samon, | 0 | 2 | 8 |
| Salte Fyche for the Coks, | 0 | 1 | 0 |
| Rydyng for Trouts | 0 | 0 | 8 |
| Mynstrels, | 0 | 16 | 0 |
| Butlers, | 0 | 1 | 6 |
| Cokys, | 0 | 17 | 4 |

FINIS.

CPSIA information can be obtained
at www.ICGtesting.com
Printed in the USA
LVHW080227080920
665307LV00011B/115